Talk to your healthcare provider about
your specific dietary restrictions.

Diabetes&Heart
HEALTHY COOKBOOK

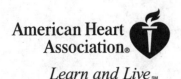

American Heart
Association®

Learn and Live sm

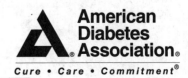

American
Diabetes
Association®

Cure • Care • Commitment®

American Diabetes Association Staff: *Director, Book Publishing,* John Fedor; *Associate Director, Consumer Books,* Sherrye Landrum; *Editor,* Laurie Guffey; *Associate Director, Book Production,* Peggy M. Rote. *Composition,* Circle Graphics; *Cover Design,* Koncept, Inc.; *Printer,* Port City Press, Inc. American Heart Association Consumer Publications Staff: *Director,* Jane Anneken Ruehl; *Senior Editor,* Janice Roth Moss; *Editor,* Jacqueline Fornerod Haigney; *Assistant Editor,* Roberta Westcott Sullivan; *Senior Marketing Manager,* Bharati Gaitonde. Recipe Developers: Linda Drachman, Nancy S. Hughes, Karen Levin, and Carol Ritchie. Cover Photo: Chicken Stir-Fry with Snow Peas and Mixed Bell Peppers, page 84.

Printed in the United States of America

5 7 9 10 8 6 4

The suggestions and information contained in this publication are generally consistent with the *Clinical Practice Recommendations* and other policies of the American Diabetes Association, but they do not represent the policy or position of the Association or any of its boards or committees. Reasonable steps have been taken to ensure the accuracy of the information presented. However, the American Diabetes Association cannot ensure the safety or efficacy of any product or service described in this publication. Individuals are advised to consult a physician or other appropriate health care professional before undertaking any diet or exercise program or taking any medication referred to in this publication. Professionals must use and apply their own professional judgment, experience, and training and should not rely solely on the information contained in this publication before prescribing any diet, exercise, or medication. The American Diabetes Association—its officers, directors, employees, volunteers, and members—assumes no responsibility or liability for personal or other injury, loss, or damage that may result from the suggestions or information in this publication.

∞ The paper in this publication meets the requirements of the ANSI Standard Z39.48-1992 (permanence of paper).

ADA titles may be purchased for business or promotional use or for special sales. To purchase this book in large quantities, or for custom editions of this book with your logo, contact Lee Romano Sequeira, Special Sales & Promotions, at the address below, or at LRomano@diabetes.org or 703-299-2046.

American Diabetes Association
1701 North Beauregard Street
Alexandria, Virginia 22311

American Heart Association
7272 Greenville Avenue
Dallas, Texas 75231

Library of Congress Cataloging-in-Publication Data

Heart healthy cookbook / American Heart Association, American Diabetes Association.
   p. cm.
   Includes index.
   ISBN 1-58040-180-5 (pbk. : alk. paper)
   1. Heart—Diseases—Diet therapy—Recipes. 2. Heart—Diseases—Prevention. I. American Heart Association. II. American Diabetes Association.

RC684.D5H437 2004
641.5'6311—dc22

            2004057543

Contents

Foreword

Into the 21st century, diabetes and heart disease continue to present a challenge. Scientific research and medical advances provide new options to treat these conditions, but the real power to improve your health and that of your family lies in the choices you make every day.

It's up to you: wise lifestyle choices, such as eating more vegetables and taking a walk every day, do reduce your risk of developing diabetes, heart disease, and stroke. If you already have diabetes or heart disease (and they go hand in hand), the choices you make will help you manage the disease.

The link between diabetes and cardiovascular disease is well established. People with diabetes are two to four times more likely than others to have heart disease or stroke. The good news, however, is that the same things that are good for diabetes are good for heart health.

The American Diabetes Association (ADA) and the American Heart Association (AHA) are proud to offer this first joint cookbook as we work together to help you live a healthier life. These taste-tested recipes were designed to follow the nutritional guidelines of both the ADA and the AHA. You can choose your meals with confidence, knowing that as you enjoy good food you are also taking care of your heart and your health.

To help you make wise choices, each recipe includes a nutritional analysis of the calories, saturated fat, cholesterol, and carbohydrate, among others. Because obesity is the leading risk factor for diabetes and a risk factor for cardiovascular disease (the most serious complication of diabetes), you are wise to eat meals that are low in calories and saturated fat. Use the analyses to tailor your eating plan to your individual needs. Remember that if you eat more calories than you burn, your weight will go up. On the other hand, if you burn more than you eat, even a little, your weight will go down.

Simple choices add up. These small steps can lead to big changes. Try to eat at least three servings of nonstarchy vegetables a day—more is even better. Try to eat two servings of fresh fruit or unsweetened frozen fruit and plenty of whole grains. Stay away from sweetened drinks (even fruit juice and milk have natural sugars, so watch your serving sizes). Drink more water. Leave the highly processed white flour, white sugar, and white fatty foods in the grocery store, and enjoy a journey through the colorful and flavorful world of fresh food prepared lightly. You'll feel so much better when you do.

Here's to your best health!

Richard Kahn, PhD
Chief Science and Medical Officer
American Diabetes Association

Rose Marie Robertson, MD, FAHA
Chief Science Officer
American Heart Association

Introduction

Eat Better, Feel Better

Diabetes is a major risk factor for heart disease and stroke. The fact is that adolescents and young adults are developing type 2 diabetes at an alarming rate. The seriousness of this situation as it relates to cardiovascular health prompted the American Heart Association and the American Diabetes Association to join forces in an effort to reverse the trend. Healthful lifestyle choices, especially appropriate diet and daily physical activity, can have a major impact on the prevention and treatment of cardiovascular disease in people with diabetes.

The American Diabetes Association and the American Heart Association want to help you make wise choices about the foods you eat. The American Heart Association has contributed to this book by developing delicious and heart-healthy recipes. These recipes are designed to be consistent with the American Diabetes Association dietary guidelines and will introduce variety into individual diabetic meal plans.

Six Simple Steps to Good Health

By following the guidelines below, you will enjoy the best of nature's bounty and, at the same time, help prevent the cardiovascular consequences of diabetes.

1. Enjoy a wide variety of foods. Eat:

   - Six or more servings of grain and whole-grain products and legumes each day.
   - Five or more servings of vegetables and fruits each day.
   - Three or more servings of fat-free or low-fat milk products for most adults, two or more for children, four for teenagers and older adults, and three to four for women who are pregnant or breastfeeding.
   - Two servings of lean meat, poultry, seafood, or vegetable protein each day. Include at least two servings of fish, especially oily fish, each week.

2. Choose a meal plan low in saturated and trans (hydrogenated) fats. Replace most of these fats with healthful polyunsaturated and monounsaturated fats.
3. Balance your food intake with physical activity to maintain a healthful weight. To lose weight, take in fewer calories or burn more until you reach a healthful goal.
4. Limit your daily intake of dietary cholesterol to less than 300 milligrams (mg).
5. Keep your intake of sodium to less than 2,400 mg per day. (If you have coronary heart disease or congestive heart failure, your doctor may recommend lower limits.)
6. If you drink alcohol, limit yourself to one drink per day if you are a woman and two drinks per day if you are a man.

What foods should be in your healthful meal plan? These serving sizes, based on the dietary exchanges from the ADA, can help you choose appropriately.

1. **Grains, Beans, and Starchy Vegetables**

   One serving =   1 slice of whole-wheat bread
   1 1/2 cups cooked oatmeal, wheat cereal, or polenta
   3/4 cup flaked cereal
   1/3 cup cooked brown rice
   1/2 cup cooked whole-grain pasta
   1/2 cup cooked legumes or starchy vegetables, such as pinto beans
   1/3 cup cooked sweet potatoes

2. **Fruits and Vegetables**

   One serving =   1 small apple, banana, orange, or pear
   1 cup cubed cantaloupe or papaya
   1 1/4 cups strawberries
   1 cup raw leafy greens
   1/2 cup cooked or chopped vegetables or fruit
   1/2 cup fruit juice or vegetable juice

3. **Meat and Meat Substitutes**

   One serving =   1 ounce fat-free or low-fat cheese
   1/2 cup fat-free or low-fat cottage cheese
   1 ounce cheese
   3 ounces cooked (4 ounces raw) lean meat, poultry, or seafood
   1/4 cup canned tuna or salmon or 3 medium sardines (packed in water)
   2 tablespoons peanut butter
   1 egg, 2 egg whites, or 1/4 cup egg substitute
   3 ounces soy product, such as tofu or soyburger

4. **Dairy Products**

   One serving =   1 cup fat-free or low-fat milk
   1 cup fat-free or low-fat yogurt

5. Fats

One serving =   10 peanuts
                     1 tablespoon sesame seeds
                     1 teaspoon margarine
                     1 teaspoon canola oil
                     2 tablespoons fat-free or low-fat sour cream

6. Other Carbohydrates

One serving =   1 granola bar
                     3 gingersnaps
                     5 vanilla wafers
               1/3 cup low-fat frozen yogurt
                     1 small brownie
               1/8 pumpkin pie

How to Use the Recipe Analyses

To help you with meal planning, we have carefully analyzed each recipe in this cookbook to provide useful nutrition information. If your healthcare professional has told you to restrict the amount of sodium or saturated fat in your meal plan, read the analyses and choose your recipes carefully.

Each analysis is based on one serving of the dish, unless otherwise indicated, and includes all the ingredients listed. Optional ingredients and garnishes, however, are not analyzed unless otherwise noted; neither are foods suggested as accompaniments.

We've made every effort to provide accurate nutrition information. Because of the many variables involved in analyzing foods, however, these values should be considered approximate.

- When a recipe lists ingredient options, such as 1/2 cup fat-free or low-fat Cheddar cheese, we analyzed the first one.
- Values except for fats are rounded to the nearest whole number. Fat values are rounded to the nearest gram. The values for saturated, monounsaturated, and polyunsaturated fats are rounded to the nearest 0.1 gram. These values may not add up to the total fat in the recipe, because total fat also includes other fatty substances and glycerol.
- We used canola oil in our recipes, but you can use any other oil with no more than 2 grams of saturated fat per tablespoon—olive, safflower, sunflower, corn, sesame, soybean, walnut, or almond.

- When selecting a stick margarine, choose one that lists liquid vegetable oil as the first ingredient. It should contain no more than 2 grams of saturated fat per tablespoon. We used corn oil stick margarine for the analysis.
- Meats are analyzed as cooked and lean, with all visible fat discarded. Values for ground beef are based on meat that is 90 percent fat free.
- After you brown ground beef without seasonings, you can wash away some of the fat by rinsing the beef under hot running water. Our recipes tell you to do this when it's practical, and this is how the beef was analyzed in those cases.
- If meat, poultry, or seafood is marinated and the marinade is discarded, we calculated only the amount of marinade absorbed. We calculated the total amount of the marinade used in marinated vegetables. We did the same for liquids used for basting or dipping.
- The specific ingredients listed in each recipe were analyzed. For instance, we used both fat-free and low-fat cream cheese in this collection of recipes, depending on the taste and texture desired. In each case, the type listed was used for the nutrition analysis. If you prefer a different variety, use it. Of course, the fat values will change with such substitutions. Other nutrient values, such as sodium, may change as well. On the other hand, if you want to substitute reconstituted lemon juice for fresh, or white onions for yellow, the substitutions won't change the ingredient analyses enough to matter.
- When no quantity is listed for an ingredient in a recipe, that ingredient cannot be figured into the analysis. For example, we don't list a quantity for the small amount of flour used to prepare a surface for kneading dough. Therefore, we don't include it in the analysis.
- We use the abbreviations "g" for gram and "mg" for milligram.

A Week of Meal Plans

You can design your own weekly meal plans using the recipes in this book. To get you started, here's a sample week from the American Diabetes Association. Keep in mind that all dishes are prepared without added salt or fats and that the dairy products used in the food preparation are fat free.

Sunday

Breakfast

  1 Lemon-Lime Poppy Seed Muffin (see page 181)
1 1/2 cups cubed cantaloupe
  1 cup fat-free milk

Morning Snack

 1/2 6-ounce carton fat-free plain yogurt
 1/2 cup fresh strawberries

Lunch

  1 serving Chicken with Country Gravy (see page 90)
 1/2 medium potato roasted in skin
  1 whole-wheat dinner roll
  1 cup mixed vegetables (no corn, peas, or pasta)
  1 tablespoon light tub margarine
 1/2 cup fat-free or low-fat ice cream

Dinner

 1/2 recipe Chunky Vegetable and Egg Salad Sandwiches (see page 148)
 3/4 cup Tomato Basil Bisque (see page 17)
  1 small apple

Evening Snack

  1 cup fat-free milk
  2 fat-free, low-sodium crispbread crackers

Monday

Breakfast

  1 serving Southwestern Breakfast Tortilla Wrap (see page 188)
 3/4 cup mixed fresh fruit
  1 cup fat-free milk

Lunch

  1 serving Tex-Mex Chili Bowl (see page 111)
  1 small apple

Afternoon Snack

   1/2 cup Apricot and Apple Granola (see page 184)

Dinner

   1/4 recipe Southwestern Pork Tenderloin Skillet (see page 121)
   1/2 cup mashed potatoes with fat-free spray margarine
    2 cups garden salad with
    1 tablespoon low-fat ranch salad dressing

Evening Snack

    1 Orange and Dried Plum Bar (see page 202)
    1 cup fat-free milk

Tuesday

Breakfast

   1/4 recipe Ham and Broccoli Frittata (see page 127)
    1 cup fat-free milk
   1/2 cup orange juice

Morning Snack

    1 Tropical Fruit and Pudding Parfait (see page 204)

Lunch

   3/4 cup Lentils with Brown Rice and Mushrooms (see page 142), mixed with
 1 1/2 ounces extra-firm light tofu
   3/4 cup mixed fresh fruit topped with
   1/2 tablespoon unsalted cashews

Afternoon Snack

   10 unsalted dry-roasted peanuts

Dinner

   1/6 recipe Slow-Cooker Swiss Steak (see page 112)
    2 cups garden salad with
    1 tablespoon balsamic vinaigrette
    1 cup cubed cantaloupe

Evening Snack

    1 Devil's Food Cupcake with Cream Cheese Topping (see page 192)
    1 cup fat-free milk

Wednesday_____

Breakfast

    1 cup French Toast Casserole with Honey-Glazed Fruit (see page 186)

    1 cup coffee

Lunch

    1/2 cup Chunky Potato Salad (see page 44)

    3 ounces fresh cooked shrimp over

    1 cup leaf lettuce, topped with

    2 tablespoons avocado and

    1 tablespoon fat-free or light Thousand Island dressing

    1 multigrain roll

    1 teaspoon light tub margarine

    3/4 cup mixed fresh fruit

Afternoon Snack

    6 ounces fat-free artificially sweetened vanilla-flavored yogurt

Dinner

    Lamb Kebabs:

    3 ounces lamb chunks

    1/2 cup onion chunks

    1/2 cup green bell pepper chunks

    1 cup tomato chunks

    1/2 cup Mediterranean Couscous with Capers (see page 161)

    17 small grapes

Evening Snack

    3 pieces Melba toast

    1 cup fat-free milk

Thursday _____

Breakfast

    Café au Lait:

    1 cup coffee

    1/2 cup fat-free milk

    2 reduced-fat crescent rolls with

    1 tablespoon sugar-free jam

    1/2 cup orange juice

Lunch

    1/12 recipe Deep-South Shrimp Gumbo (see page 79)
        2 ounces sliced beef tenderloin on
        1 small hoagie roll with
      1/4 cup canned fat-free gravy and
      1/4 cup chopped lettuce and
      1/4 cup chopped tomato

Dinner

        3 ounces grilled catfish
      1/8 recipe Red Beans and Brown Rice (see page 137)
      3/4 cup mixed fresh fruit topped with
        3 dry-roasted unsalted almonds, chopped

Evening Snack

        6 ounces fat-free artificially sweetened vanilla-flavored yogurt

Friday

Breakfast

        1 cup cooked oatmeal mixed with
        6 dry-roasted unsalted sliced almonds and
        2 tablespoons raisins
        1 cup fat-free milk

Lunch

    1 1/4 cups Corn and Ham Chowder (see page 25)
        1 open-face cheese sandwich:
        1 slice whole-wheat bread
        1 ounce provolone cheese
        2 tablespoons chopped avocado
      1/4 cup chopped tomato
      1/4 cup chopped lettuce
        1 small apple

Afternoon Snack

        1 Lemon-Lime Poppy Seed Muffin (see page 181)

Dinner

        3 ounces cooked halibut
      2/3 cup cooked brown rice with fat-free spray margarine
        1 cup Farmer's Market Veggie Salad (see page 41)
        1 cup fat-free milk

Evening Snack
> 3/4 cup Chocolate-Mocha Cooler (see page 13)

Saturday

Breakfast
> 1 piece Apple Crumble Coffee Cake (see page 182)
> 3/4 cup mixed fresh fruit
> 1 cup fat-free milk

Morning Snack
> 1 slice Rosemary and Dill Quick Bread (see page 180)

Lunch
> 1/4 recipe Tuna-Macaroni Casserole with Tomatoes and Chickpeas (see page 69)
> 1/2 fresh pear
> 4 walnut halves

Afternoon Snack
> Snack mix:
> 1/3 cup thin pretzel sticks
> 5 unsalted dry-roasted peanuts
> 1 tablespoon raisins

Dinner
> 3 ounces cooked pork tenderloin
> 1 cup Crunchy Asian Snow Pea Salad (see page 38)
> 1/2 cup cooked corn
> 1 whole-wheat dinner roll
> 2 teaspoons light tub margarine
> 1 1/4 cup cubed watermelon

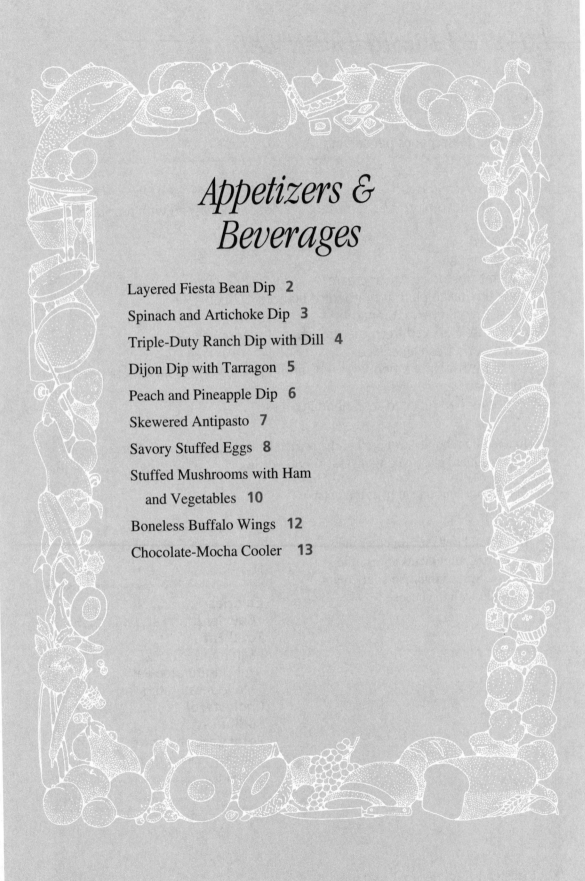

Appetizers & Beverages

Layered Fiesta Bean Dip

Zesty pico de gallo updates a party classic.

Serves 20; 2 tablespoons per serving

1/2 16-ounce can no-salt-added low-fat refried beans or 1/2 15-ounce can no-salt-added pinto beans, rinsed, drained, and mashed with a potato masher
1/4 cup salsa
1/8 teaspoon salt
1/2 cup fat-free or light sour cream
1 medium Italian plum tomato, diced (about 1/2 cup)
1/4 small onion, finely chopped
1/8 cup loosely packed fresh cilantro, coarsely chopped
1/2 tablespoon fresh lime juice
1/2 small fresh jalapeño pepper, seeds and ribs discarded, coarsely chopped (optional)
1/4 cup shredded reduced-fat Cheddar cheese

1 In a medium bowl, stir together the refried beans, salsa, and salt. Spread in an 8-inch square glass baking dish or serving dish.

2 Spread the sour cream over the bean mixture.

3 In a small bowl, stir together the remaining ingredients except the cheese. Spread over the sour cream. Sprinkle with the cheese.

EXCHANGES

Free Food

Calories 23
Calories from Fat 5
Total Fat .... 1 g
Saturated Fat .... 0.2 g
Polyunsaturated Fat .... 0.1 g
Monounsaturated Fat ..... 0.2 g
Cholesterol .... 2 mg
Sodium .... 44 mg
Total Carbohydrate .... 4 g
Dietary Fiber .... 1 g
Sugars .... 1 g
Protein .... 1 g

Spinach and Artichoke Dip

A captivating blend of artichokes, spinach, sour cream, and aromatic flavorings makes every bite of this dip memorable.

Serves 26; 2 tablespoons per serving

14-ounce can artichoke heart quarters, rinsed and drained, chopped
10 ounces frozen chopped spinach, thawed and squeezed dry
1 1/2 cups fat-free or light sour cream
1/2 cup chopped roasted red bell peppers, rinsed and drained if bottled
1/2 cup shredded Parmesan cheese
2 medium green onions, thinly sliced (green and white parts)
1 tablespoon dried onion flakes or 1 teaspoon onion powder
1 teaspoon prepared white horseradish (optional)
1/2 teaspoon garlic powder
1/8 teaspoon red hot-pepper sauce

In a medium bowl, stir together all the ingredients. Refrigerate for at least 30 minutes, or until the onion flakes have softened.

EXCHANGES

1 Vegetable

Calories	27
Calories from Fat	6
Total Fat	1 g
Saturated Fat	0.3 g
Polyunsaturated Fat	0.1 g
Monounsaturated Fat	0.2 g
Cholesterol	2 mg
Sodium	75 mg
Total Carbohydrate	4 g
Dietary Fiber	0 g
Sugars	1 g
Protein	2 g

Triple-Duty Ranch Dip with Dill

Dunk all kinds of fresh, crisp vegetables into this cool and refreshing dip, or use it as a salad dressing or even a sauce for salmon.

Serves 16; 2 tablespoons per serving

  1   cup fat-free or low-fat buttermilk
  1   cup fat-free or light sour cream
  1   tablespoon snipped fresh dill weed or 1 teaspoon dried dill weed, crumbled
  1   tablespoon chopped green onion (green part only)
  1   tablespoon snipped fresh parsley or 1 teaspoon dried parsley, crumbled
  1   teaspoon onion powder
1/2   teaspoon garlic powder
1/2   teaspoon dry mustard
1/2   teaspoon coarsely ground pepper
1/4   teaspoon salt

In a medium bowl, whisk together all the ingredients. Cover and refrigerate for at least 30 minutes before serving.

EXCHANGES

Free Food

Calories	21
Calories from Fat	1
Total Fat	0 g
Saturated Fat	0 g
Polyunsaturated Fat	0 g
Monounsaturated Fat	0 g
Cholesterol	2 mg
Sodium	71 mg
Total Carbohydrate	4 g
Dietary Fiber	0 g
Sugars	2 g
Protein	1 g

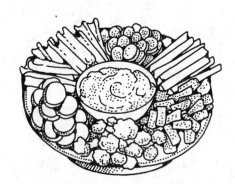

Dijon Dip with Tarragon

Precut vegetables, such as celery and broccoli, make good dippers for this quick dip.

Serves 6; 2 tablespoons per serving

    1/2 cup fat-free or light sour cream
      2 tablespoons fat-free or light mayonnaise dressing
      2 tablespoons Dijon mustard
      2 teaspoons olive oil (extra virgin preferred)
  1 1/4 teaspoons dried tarragon, crumbled
    1/2 medium garlic clove, minced
    1/4 teaspoon salt

In a small bowl, whisk together all the ingredients until smooth.

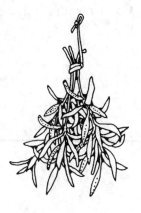

EXCHANGES

1/2 Carbohydrate

Calories 40
  Calories from Fat 15
Total Fat...........................2 g
  Saturated Fat ....0.2 g
  Polyunsaturated Fat ....0.2 g
  Monounsaturated Fat .....1.2 g
Cholesterol ....1 mg
Sodium..........................276 mg
Total Carbohydrate...........5 g
  Dietary Fiber ....0 g
  Sugars ....2 g
Protein ....1 g

Peach and Pineapple Dip

For a double dose of ginger, try reduced-fat gingersnaps with this ginger-enhanced dip. It's great for a party or to keep on hand to satisfy your sweet tooth in a heart healthy way.

Serves 20; 2 tablespoons per serving

    15-ounce can light sliced peaches in extra-light syrup, drained
1   cup drained pineapple chunks canned in their own juice
8   ounces fat-free or reduced-fat cream cheese, softened
1   tablespoon honey
1/4 teaspoon ground ginger
1/8 teaspoon ground nutmeg
1/2 cup drained mandarin oranges canned in water

1 In a food processor or blender, process all the ingredients except the mandarin oranges to the desired texture (either smooth or slightly chunky).

2 To serve, put the spread in a large shallow bowl. Garnish with the mandarin oranges.

EXCHANGES

1/2 Fruit

Calories	27
Calories from Fat	0
Total Fat	0 g
Saturated Fat	0 g
Polyunsaturated Fat	0 g
Monounsaturated Fat	0 g
Cholesterol	1 mg
Sodium	61 mg
Total Carbohydrate	5 g
Dietary Fiber	0 g
Sugars	4 g
Protein	2 g

Skewered Antipasto

Entertaining doesn't need to be difficult. Treat your guests to these impressive but easy appetizers. (See photo insert.)

Serves 8; 1 skewer per serving

8 baby spinach leaves
8 grape tomatoes or cherry tomatoes
8 small pitted ripe olives
2 ounces fat-free or part-skim mozzarella cheese, cut into 8 1/2-inch cubes
2 canned artichokes, quartered, rinsed, and drained
2 canned hearts of palm stalks, each cut crosswise into 4 pieces, rinsed, and drained
8 turkey pepperoni slices
2 tablespoons balsamic vinegar
2 teaspoons olive oil (extra virgin preferred)
1 teaspoon dried basil, crumbled
1/2 teaspoon dried oregano, crumbled

1 Thread a 6-inch skewer with 1 each spinach leaf, grape tomato, olive, cheese cube, artichoke heart quarter, heart of palm piece, and pepperoni slice. Repeat with seven more skewers. Place on a platter.

2 In a small bowl, whisk together the remaining ingredients. Spoon evenly over the skewers.

EXCHANGES

1 Lean Meat

Calories	41
Calories from Fat	17
Total Fat	2 g
Saturated Fat	0.3 g
Polyunsaturated Fat	0.2 g
Monounsaturated Fat	1.2 g
Cholesterol	3 mg
Sodium	171 mg
Total Carbohydrate	3 g
Dietary Fiber	1 g
Sugars	1 g
Protein	3 g

COOK'S TIP

If you prefer, omit the skewers, instead arranging the ingredients in a single layer on the platter and topping with the dressing. Use wooden picks to spear the food, if desired.

Savory Stuffed Eggs

Double the filling options for double the appetizer fun! Hard-cooked egg whites are the perfect canvas for two different but complementary savory fillings. If you prefer to stuff all the eggs with only one of the fillings, double the ingredients for that filling and proceed as directed below.

Serves 12; 2 stuffed halves per serving

12 large hard-cooked eggs, peeled

SALMON FILLING
6-ounce can red or pink salmon, drained, bones discarded if desired and skin discarded
1 tablespoon fat-free or reduced-fat mayonnaise dressing
1 tablespoon dill-pickle relish
1 teaspoon Dijon mustard
1 teaspoon fresh lemon juice

BEAN FILLING
1/2 cup canned no-salt-added kidney beans, rinsed and drained
1/4 cup salsa
2 tablespoons chopped black olives
1/2 teaspoon ground cumin
1/4 teaspoon salt

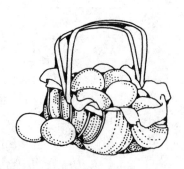

1 Slice the eggs in half lengthwise. Remove and discard the yolks. Place the whites with the inside up on a platter.

2 In a medium bowl, stir together the salmon filling ingredients. Spoon about 1/2 tablespoon filling into each of 12 egg white halves.

3 For the bean filling, in a second medium bowl, mash the beans with a potato masher. Stir in the remaining ingredients. Spoon about 1/2 tablespoon filling into each of the remaining 12 egg white halves.

COOK'S TIP

Drain the water from the pot in which you cooked the eggs. Pour in cold water to cover the eggs. Pressing lightly, roll each egg on a flat surface, such as a countertop, so the shells crack into many small pieces. Hold each egg under cold running water and peel from the wider end. The water makes it easier to peel the eggs and rinses off any bits of shell that you miss.

EXCHANGES

1 Lean Meat

Calories	49
Calories from Fat	10
Total Fat	1 g
Saturated Fat	0.2 g
Polyunsaturated Fat	0.3 g
Monounsaturated Fat	0.5 g
Cholesterol	5 mg
Sodium	224 mg
Total Carbohydrate	3 g
Dietary Fiber	1 g
Sugars	1 g
Protein	7 g

Stuffed Mushrooms with Ham and Vegetables

Every bite of these mushroom morsels is packed with flavor from fresh veggies and moist ham and with texture from crunchy walnuts.

Serves 8; 4 mushrooms per serving

```
   1  slice whole-wheat bread (about 1 ounce)
  32  small button mushrooms (about 1 pound)
      Vegetable oil spray
   1  medium carrot, shredded
   2  ounces lower-sodium, low-fat ham, diced (about 1/4 cup)
 1/4  cup shredded Parmesan cheese
      Egg substitute equivalent to 1 egg, or 1 large egg
   2  tablespoons chopped walnuts
   1  medium green onion, finely chopped (green and white parts)
   1  tablespoon chili sauce
```

> **COOK'S TIP**
>
> *When you crave a quick, bite-size snack, marinate 1 pound of mushrooms in 1/4 cup of your favorite low-sodium, fat-free or reduced-fat vinaigrette. The marinated mushrooms will keep in an airtight container in the refrigerator for up to three days.*

1 Toast the bread until golden brown. Let cool. Dice.

2 Preheat the oven to 350°F.

3 Remove and save the stems from the mushrooms. Put the mushroom caps with the stem side down on a large nonstick baking sheet. Lightly spray the tops with vegetable oil spray. Turn the mushrooms over.

4 Finely chop the stems. Put the chopped stems in a medium bowl. Stir the remaining ingredients into the chopped stems. Spoon about 2 teaspoons mixture into the cavity of each mushroom.

5 Bake, uncovered, for 25 to 30 minutes, or until the mushrooms are tender and the filling is warmed through.

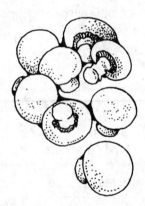

EXCHANGES

1/2 Fat
1/2 Carbohydrate

Calories	65
Calories from Fat	23
Total Fat	3 g
Saturated Fat	0.6 g
Polyunsaturated Fat	0.9 g
Monounsaturated Fat	0.7 g
Cholesterol	6 mg
Sodium	144 mg
Total Carbohydrate	7 g
Dietary Fiber	1 g
Sugars	2 g
Protein	5 g

Boneless Buffalo Wings

Boneless chicken breast meat stands in for traditional chicken wings in this easy-to-prepare recipe. An enhanced barbecue sauce is tossed with the baked chicken to make it even more lip-smackin' good!

Serves 14; 2 pieces chicken and scant 1/2 tablespoon sauce per serving

Vegetable oil spray
2 tablespoons whole-wheat flour or all-purpose flour
1/4 teaspoon salt-free seasoned pepper blend
1 pound boneless, skinless chicken breasts, all visible fat discarded
1/4 cup fat-free or low-fat buttermilk
1 teaspoon red hot-pepper sauce
1 cup crushed cornflake cereal (about 2 1/2 cups flakes)
1/4 cup barbecue sauce
1 tablespoon cider vinegar
1 tablespoon honey

1 Preheat the oven to 350°F. Lightly spray a baking sheet with vegetable oil spray.

2 In a large airtight plastic bag, stir together the flour and seasoned pepper blend. Cut the chicken into 28 strips. Add to the flour mixture. Seal the bag and shake to coat.

3 Add the buttermilk and hot-pepper sauce. Reseal the bag and shake gently to coat.

4 Put the cornflake crumbs in a shallow bowl. Add the chicken, turning gently to coat. Arrange the chicken in a single layer on the baking sheet. Lightly spray the chicken with vegetable oil spray.

5 Bake, uncovered, for about 25 minutes, or until the chicken is no longer pink in the center and the coating is crispy.

6 Meanwhile, in a medium bowl, stir together the barbecue sauce, vinegar, and honey.

7 Add the chicken to the sauce, stirring gently to coat, or serve the sauce on the side.

EXCHANGES

1/2 Starch
1 Very Lean Meat

Calories 74
  Calories from Fat 9
Total Fat...........................1 g
  Saturated Fat ....0.3 g
  Polyunsaturated Fat ....0.2 g
  Monounsaturated Fat .....0.3 g
Cholesterol ....20 mg
Sodium...........................127 mg
Total Carbohydrate...........8 g
  Dietary Fiber ....0 g
  Sugars ....3 g
Protein ....8 g

Chocolate-Mocha Cooler

There's something about coffee that perks up the already-marvelous flavor of chocolate. One sip of this creamy, icy-cold drink will make our point.

Serves 4; 3/4 cup per serving

  1 cup fat-free milk
  2 cups frozen fat-free or reduced-fat chocolate ice cream
  2 tablespoons packed dark brown sugar
  1 tablespoon instant coffee granules
  2 teaspoons vanilla extract
1/4 teaspoon peppermint extract
  1 to 2 tablespoons coffee-flavored liqueur (optional)

Put all the ingredients in a blender in the order listed. Blend until smooth. Serve immediately.

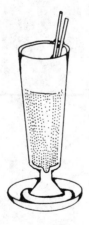

EXCHANGES

2 Carbohydrate

Calories	146
Calories from Fat	15
Total Fat	2 g
Saturated Fat	1.1 g
Polyunsaturated Fat	0 g
Monounsaturated Fat	0.4 g
Cholesterol	6 mg
Sodium	70 mg
Total Carbohydrate	31 g
Dietary Fiber	4 g
Sugars	24 g
Protein	5 g

Soups

Broccoli Cheese Soup   16

Tomato Basil Bisque   17

Creamy Caramelized Onion Soup   18

Loaded Baked Potato Soup   20

Split Pea and Lima Bean Soup with Chicken   22

Home-Style Vegetable Beef Soup   23

Pork, Barley, and Vegetable Stew   24

Corn and Ham Chowder   25

Mushroom and Barley Stew   26

Vegetable Stew with Fresh Rosemary   28

Italian Lentil Soup   30

Broccoli Cheese Soup

If you enjoy broccoli cheese soup at restaurants, you will be pleased to know how easy it is to make a delectable, healthful version at home.

Serves 8; 3/4 cup per serving

1 teaspoon canola oil
1 small onion, finely chopped
2 medium garlic cloves, minced
2 cups low-fat, low-sodium chicken broth
1 pound broccoli florets, chopped (about 4 cups)
1/2 teaspoon dry mustard
1/4 teaspoon salt
1/4 teaspoon pepper
1/8 teaspoon red hot-pepper sauce (optional)
2 cups fat-free milk
1/3 cup all-purpose flour
1/2 cup fat-free half-and-half
2 ounces fat-free or reduced-fat Cheddar cheese, sliced or shredded
2 tablespoons shredded Parmesan cheese

1 Heat a large saucepan over medium heat. Pour the oil into the pan and swirl to coat the bottom. Cook the onion and garlic for 3 to 4 minutes, or until the onion is tender.

2 Stir in the broth, broccoli, mustard, salt, pepper, and hot-pepper sauce. Increase the heat to medium high and bring to a simmer. Reduce the heat and simmer, uncovered, for 5 minutes, or until the broccoli is tender, stirring occasionally.

3 In a medium bowl, whisk together the milk and flour. Stir into the soup. Simmer for 2 to 3 minutes, or until the mixture has thickened, stirring occasionally.

4 Stir in the remaining ingredients. Cook over medium-low heat for 1 to 2 minutes, or until the cheeses have melted, stirring occasionally.

EXCHANGES

1/2 Fat
1 Carbohydrate

Calories 97
 Calories from Fat 18
Total Fat .... 2 g
 Saturated Fat .... 0.6 g
 Polyunsaturated Fat .... 0.4 g
 Monounsaturated Fat ..... 0.6 g
Cholesterol .... 5 mg
Sodium .... 226 mg
Total Carbohydrate .... 13 g
 Dietary Fiber .... 1 g
 Sugars .... 6 g
Protein .... 8 g

Tomato Basil Bisque

Fresh basil gives a blast of flavor to every spoonful of this soup, whether served warm or chilled.

Serves 8; 3/4 cup per serving

1/2 cup low-fat, low-sodium chicken broth
2 medium leeks (white part only), thinly sliced, or 1/2 cup sliced onion
1 small rib of celery, diced
2 medium garlic cloves, minced
1/4 teaspoon salt

1/4 teaspoon pepper
2 pounds large tomatoes (about 4)
1/2 cup low-fat, low-sodium chicken broth
1/4 cup fresh basil, loosely packed
1/2 cup fat-free half-and-half

1   In a medium saucepan, stir together 1/2 cup broth, leeks, celery, garlic, salt, and pepper. Bring to a simmer over medium-high heat. Reduce the heat and simmer, covered, for 5 minutes, or until the vegetables are tender. Remove from the heat and let cool for 5 minutes.

2   Pour the broth mixture into a food processor or blender. Process for about 1 minute, or until smooth. Return the mixture to the saucepan. Keep warm over low heat (uncovered).

3   Fill a small saucepan half-full with cold water. Bring to a boil over high heat. Reduce the heat to medium high. Cut a small *X* on the bottom of each tomato so the skin will loosen more easily. Put 2 tomatoes in the saucepan. Simmer for 10 seconds, or until the peel starts to loosen from the flesh. Transfer to a cutting board. Repeat with the remaining tomatoes. Let the tomatoes cool for a few minutes. Remove the peel if desired. Cut the tomatoes into quarters.

4   In a food processor or blender, process the tomatoes and the remaining 1/2 cup broth in batches until smooth, about 1 minute per batch. Before processing the last batch, add the basil.

5   Pour the tomato mixture into the leek mixture. Increase the heat to medium high and bring to a simmer. Reduce the heat and simmer, partially covered, for 8 to 10 minutes, or until the flavors have blended, stirring occasionally.

6   Stir in the half-and-half. Cook over low heat for 1 to 2 minutes, or until the mixture is warmed through, stirring occasionally. Serve warm or refrigerate in an airtight container until chilled.

EXCHANGES

1/2 Carbohydrate

Calories	43
Calories from Fat	7
Total Fat	1 g
Saturated Fat	0.2 g
Polyunsaturated Fat	0.2 g
Monounsaturated Fat	0.1 g
Cholesterol	2 mg
Sodium	121 mg
Total Carbohydrate	8 g
Dietary Fiber	1 g
Sugars	4 g
Protein	2 g

Creamy Caramelized Onion Soup

A bowl of this creamy version of onion soup with a spinach and lean ham salad makes a nice lunch.

Serves 8; 3/4 cup per serving

- 2 6-inch whole-wheat pita breads
- 1 teaspoon olive oil
- 2 large onions, thinly sliced
- 1/4 teaspoon salt
- 1/4 teaspoon sugar
- 2 medium garlic cloves, minced
- 4 cups low-fat, low-sodium chicken broth
- 1/4 teaspoon pepper
- 1 cup fat-free half-and-half
- 1/3 cup all-purpose flour
- 3 tablespoons shredded Parmesan cheese

COOK'S TIP

You can store the toasted pita triangles at room temperature in an airtight container for up to five days.

1 Preheat the oven to 375°F.

2 Cut each pita bread into 6 triangles. Separate the tops from the bottoms (you will have 24 triangles total). Arrange the triangles in a single layer on a large nonstick baking sheet.

3 Bake for 8 to 10 minutes, or until crisp. Transfer the baking sheet to a cooling rack. Set aside to cool for at least 15 minutes.

4 Heat a large saucepan over medium-high heat. Pour the oil into the pan and swirl to coat the bottom. Cook the onions for 2 minutes, stirring occasionally.

5 Stir in the salt and sugar. Cook for 7 to 10 minutes, or until the onions are a deep, golden brown, stirring occasionally.

6 Stir in the garlic. Cook for 30 seconds, or until tender, stirring occasionally. Stir in the broth and pepper. Bring to a simmer. Reduce the heat and simmer for 10 minutes, or until the onions are tender and the flavors have blended.

7 In a medium bowl, whisk together the half-and-half and flour. Pour into the soup mixture. Increase the heat to medium high. Cook for 3 to 4 minutes, or until the mixture has thickened, stirring occasionally.

8 To serve, ladle the soup into bowls. Top each serving with 3 pita triangles and about 1 teaspoon Parmesan cheese.

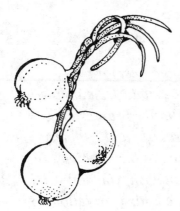

EXCHANGES

1/2 Fat
1 1/2 Carbohydrate

Calories	134
Calories from Fat	25
Total Fat	3 g
Saturated Fat	0.9 g
Polyunsaturated Fat	0.4 g
Monounsaturated Fat	0.9 g
Cholesterol	6 mg
Sodium	272 mg
Total Carbohydrate	21 g
Dietary Fiber	2 g
Sugars	6 g
Protein	6 g

Loaded Baked Potato Soup

This rich-tasting soup is bursting with the flavor of a baked potato and all the trimmings.

Serves 8; 3/4 cup per serving

1 1/2   pounds baking potatoes (russet preferred)
   3   cups low-fat, low-sodium chicken broth
   2   tablespoons imitation bacon bits
   1   teaspoon onion powder
1/2   teaspoon garlic powder
1/4   teaspoon salt
1/4   teaspoon pepper
   1   cup fat-free half-and-half
   3   tablespoons all-purpose flour
   2   tablespoons sliced green onions (green part only)
1/3   cup shredded fat-free or reduced-fat Cheddar cheese
1/3   cup fat-free or light sour cream

COOK'S TIP

To enhance mashed potatoes, for every 4 cups cooked potatoes, add 1/2 cup low-fat, low-sodium chicken broth, 1 tablespoon prepared white horseradish, and 2 tablespoons chopped fresh herbs, such as basil, chives, or dill. Mash as usual. If you wish, you can substitute 3 cups of potatoes prepared this way, leftover mashed potatoes prepared in a heart-healthy way, or mashed potatoes from the refrigerated section of your grocery for the 1 1/2 pounds of potatoes in this soup.

1 Preheat the oven to 350°F.

2 Pierce each potato several times with a fork. Put the potatoes on a baking sheet.

3 Bake for 1 hour, or until tender when pierced with a fork or knife.

4 Let the potatoes cool for at least 10 minutes. Peel the potatoes or cut the potatoes in half and scoop out the flesh. Put the potatoes or the scooped-out flesh in a medium saucepan. Mash with a potato masher until slightly chunky.

5 Stir in the broth, bacon bits, onion powder, garlic powder, salt, and pepper. Bring to a simmer over medium-high heat. Reduce the heat and simmer, covered, for 6 to 8 minutes, or until the flavors have blended, stirring occasionally.

6 In a medium bowl, whisk together the half-and-half and flour. Whisk into the potato mixture along with the green onions. Increase the heat to medium high and bring to a simmer. Reduce the heat and simmer, uncovered, for 2 to 3 minutes, or until the mixture has thickened.

7 To serve, ladle into bowls. Top each serving with the cheese and sour cream.

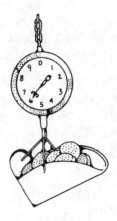

EXCHANGES

1 1/2 Carbohydrate

Calories	114
Calories from Fat	12
Total Fat	1 g
Saturated Fat	0.4 g
Polyunsaturated Fat	0.3 g
Monounsaturated Fat	0.2 g
Cholesterol	5 mg
Sodium	244 mg
Total Carbohydrate	19 g
Dietary Fiber	1 g
Sugars	4 g
Protein	6 g

Split Pea and Lima Bean Soup with Chicken

This tasty soup boasts tender chunks of chicken and plump baby carrots in a hearty base of split peas and lima beans. Serve with a crisp salad of mixed lettuces and juicy tomatoes.

Serves 6; 1 1/2 cups per serving

- 4 cups water
- 2 cups low-fat, low-sodium chicken broth
- 1 cup dried split peas, sorted for stones and shriveled peas and rinsed
- 1 pound boneless, skinless chicken breasts, all visible fat discarded, cut into 3/4-inch cubes
- 15-ounce can no-salt-added lima beans, rinsed and drained, or 1 3/4 cups frozen lima beans
- 2 cups baby carrots
- 2 medium ribs of celery, cut into 1/2-inch slices
- 2 tablespoons imitation bacon bits
- 2 teaspoons onion powder
- 1 teaspoon dried thyme, crumbled
- 1 teaspoon dried marjoram, crumbled
- 1/2 teaspoon salt
- 1/4 teaspoon pepper

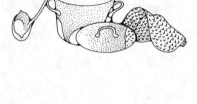

EXCHANGES

2 Starch
3 Very Lean Meat

Calories	270
Calories from Fat	29
Total Fat	3 g
Saturated Fat	0.8 g
Polyunsaturated Fat	0.9 g
Monounsaturated Fat	0.9 g
Cholesterol	46 mg
Sodium	348 mg
Total Carbohydrate	32 g
Dietary Fiber	11 g
Sugars	6 g
Protein	29 g

1 In a stockpot or Dutch oven, bring the water, broth, and peas to a boil over high heat, stirring occasionally. Reduce the heat and simmer, covered, for 45 minutes, or until the peas are almost tender (no stirring needed).

2 Stir in the remaining ingredients. Simmer, covered, for 30 to 40 minutes, or until the peas and carrots are tender and the chicken is cooked through, stirring occasionally.

Home-Style Vegetable Beef Soup

This soup freezes well, so you may want to make a double batch. Then, when you are short on time and want a home-cooked meal, you have a backup ready to heat and eat.

Serves 8; 1 1/2 cups per serving

2 pounds boneless eye of round, all visible fat discarded, cut into 1/2-inch cubes
4 cups fat-free, no-salt-added beef broth
2 cups water
  14.5-ounce can no-salt-added diced tomatoes, undrained
1 pound red potatoes, cut into 3/4-inch cubes
2 medium carrots, cut into 1/2-inch slices
1 cup diced cauliflower
1 cup fresh, frozen, or no-salt-added canned whole-kernel corn, rinsed if desired and drained if canned
1 medium onion, diced
1 tablespoon low-sodium Worcestershire sauce
1 teaspoon dried thyme, crumbled
1 teaspoon dried oregano, crumbled
1/2 teaspoon salt
1/4 teaspoon pepper

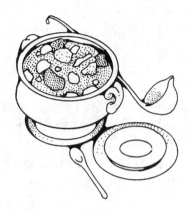

1 In a large stockpot or Dutch oven, stir together the beef, broth, water, and undrained tomatoes. Bring to a boil over high heat. Reduce the heat and simmer, covered, for 45 minutes, or until the beef is starting to get tender (no stirring needed).

2 Stir in the remaining ingredients. Simmer, covered, for 30 minutes, or until the vegetables and beef are tender, stirring occasionally.

EXCHANGES

1 Starch
3 Very Lean Meat
1 Vegetable
1/2 Fat

Calories 235
  Calories from Fat 38
Total Fat............................4 g
  Saturated Fat ....1.4 g
  Polyunsaturated Fat ....0.3 g
  Monounsaturated Fat .....1.7 g
Cholesterol ....57 mg
Sodium...........................301 mg
Total Carbohydrate.........22 g
  Dietary Fiber ....4 g
  Sugars ....6 g
Protein ....28 g

Pork, Barley, and Vegetable Stew

A bowl of this stew is very satisfying, especially during the winter months. It packs in lean pork, hearty barley, and a variety of vegetables, including vitamin-rich greens.

Serves 4; 2 cups per serving

  6 cups low-fat, low-sodium chicken broth
  1 pound boneless pork loin chops, all visible fat discarded, cut into 3/4-inch cubes
  1 teaspoon ground cumin
1/4 teaspoon pepper
  4 cups coarsely chopped collard greens or kale (about 1-inch pieces)
  1 cup baby carrots
  1 cup frozen pearl onions
  2 medium ribs of celery, cut into 1/2-inch slices
1/2 cup uncooked pearl barley
  2 tablespoons imitation bacon bits
  2 medium garlic cloves, minced

1 In a stockpot or Dutch oven, stir together the broth, pork, cumin, and pepper. Bring to a boil over high heat. Reduce the heat and simmer, covered, for 30 minutes, or until the pork is cooked through, stirring occasionally.

2 Stir in the remaining ingredients. Simmer, covered, for 30 to 35 minutes, or until the barley, vegetables, and pork are tender, stirring occasionally.

EXCHANGES

1 Starch
4 Lean Meat
2 Vegetable

Calories 327
  Calories from Fat 87
Total Fat...........................10 g
  Saturated Fat ....2.8 g
  Polyunsaturated Fat ....1.8 g
  Monounsaturated Fat .....3.6 g
Cholesterol ....68 mg
Sodium...........................303 mg
Total Carbohydrate.........27 g
  Dietary Fiber ....5 g
  Sugars ....7 g
Protein ....34 g

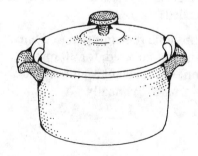

Corn and Ham Chowder

Pair this creamy, chunky chowder with a vegetable slaw and a whole-wheat muffin for Sunday supper.

Serves 4; 1 1/4 cups per serving

Vegetable oil spray
1 teaspoon canola oil
1/2 cup chopped onion
1 small rib of celery, chopped
2 tablespoons imitation bacon bits
2 cups low-fat, low-sodium chicken broth
15-ounce can no-salt-added cream-style corn, undrained

1 cup frozen whole-kernel corn or kernels from 1 large ear of grilled corn (see Cook's Tip, below)
3 ounces low-fat, lower-sodium ham, diced (about 1/2 cup)
1/8 teaspoon salt
1/4 teaspoon pepper (white preferred)
1/2 cup fat-free half-and-half
1/4 cup all-purpose flour

COOK'S TIP

For an even more flavorful soup, fire up your grill. Put one large husked and desilked ear of corn over medium-high heat. Cook, covered, for about 4 minutes, or until the corn is cooked through and slightly caramelized, turning at 1-minute intervals. Cool for about 5 minutes. Slice the kernels off the cob.

1 Heat a medium saucepan over medium heat. Remove from the heat and lightly coat with vegetable oil spray (being careful not to spray near a gas flame). Pour in the oil and swirl to coat the bottom. Cook the onion and celery for 2 to 3 minutes, or until the onion is tender, stirring occasionally.

2 Stir in the bacon bits. Cook for 1 minute, or until they are slightly rehydrated.

3 Stir in the broth, undrained cream-style corn, whole-kernel corn, ham, salt, and pepper. Increase the heat to medium high and bring to a simmer. Reduce the heat and simmer, covered, for 6 to 8 minutes, or until the flavors have blended, stirring occasionally.

4 In a medium bowl, whisk together the half-and-half and flour. Whisk into the corn mixture. Simmer, uncovered, for 3 to 4 minutes, or until the mixture has thickened and the flour doesn't taste raw.

EXCHANGES

2 Starch
1 Lean Meat

Calories 201
Calories from Fat 39
Total Fat.............................4 g
Saturated Fat ....0.8 g
Polyunsaturated Fat ....1.1 g
Monounsaturated Fat .....1.4 g
Cholesterol ....14 mg
Sodium..........................404 mg
Total Carbohydrate.........33 g
Dietary Fiber ....4 g
Sugars ....11 g
Protein ....10 g

Mushroom and Barley Stew

Chock-full of vegetables, including three varieties of mushroom, this stew is deep, rich, and intense in flavor.

Serves 4; 1 1/2 cups per serving

1/3 cup uncooked pearl barley
  2 teaspoons canola oil
  1 medium onion, chopped
  1 medium carrot, chopped
  1 small parsnip, peeled and chopped
1/2 small green, red, or yellow bell pepper, chopped
  1 medium rib of celery, chopped
  2 medium garlic cloves, crushed or minced
  3 ounces button mushrooms, chopped
  3 ounces cremini (brown) mushrooms, chopped
     14.5-ounce can no-salt-added diced tomatoes, undrained
  2 cups reduced-sodium vegetable broth or 1 cup broth and 1 cup water
1/4 ounce dried oyster or porcini mushrooms, snipped
1/4 teaspoon salt
1/4 teaspoon pepper
  1 tablespoon chopped fresh thyme or 1 teaspoon dried thyme, crumbled

> **COOK'S TIP**
>
> *A good source of vitamin C, parsnips are root vegetables related to carrots. Buy parsnips 7 to 8 inches long. If you buy larger ones, they will be more likely to have woody cores. Store parsnips in perforated plastic bags in the crisper section of your refrigerator for up to three weeks. Parsnips are almost always eaten cooked, whether steamed, baked, boiled, or microwaved. Peel parsnips before eating them.*

1 Cook the barley using the package directions, omitting the salt.

2 Heat a large nonstick saucepan over medium heat. Pour the oil into the saucepan and swirl to coat the bottom. Cook the onion, carrot, parsnip, bell pepper, celery, and garlic for 8 to 10 minutes, or until the parsnip is tender, stirring occasionally.

3 Stir in the button and cremini mushrooms. Cook for 2 to 4 minutes, or until they begin to soften, stirring occasionally.

4 Stir in the remaining ingredients. Increase the heat to high and bring to a boil. Stir in the barley. Reduce the heat and simmer, covered, for 10 minutes, stirring occasionally.

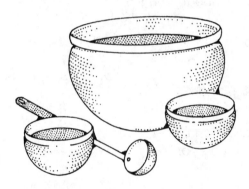

EXCHANGES

1/2 Starch
3 Vegetable
1/2 Fat

Calories	143
Calories from Fat	23
Total Fat	3 g
Saturated Fat	0.2 g
Polyunsaturated Fat	0.8 g
Monounsaturated Fat	1.4 g
Cholesterol	0 mg
Sodium	387 mg
Total Carbohydrate	28 g
Dietary Fiber	6 g
Sugars	8 g
Protein	4 g

Vegetable Stew with Fresh Rosemary

If you have a green thumb or enjoy visiting farmers' markets, feel free to create new combinations based on the freshest vegetables and herbs available. (See Cook's Tip, below, for some ideas.)

Serves 4; 1 1/2 cups per serving

  3 cups low-fat, low-sodium chicken broth
  8 small red potatoes, halved (about 8 ounces)
  1 cup baby carrots
1/2 cup frozen pearl onions
  1 small zucchini, diced (about 4 ounces)
  1 medium yellow summer squash, diced (about 4 ounces)
  4 ounces sliced button mushrooms
  1 tablespoon chopped fresh rosemary or 1 teaspoon dried rosemary, crushed
1/2 teaspoon salt
1/4 teaspoon pepper
  1 cup low-fat, low-sodium chicken broth
1/3 cup all-purpose flour
  8 ounces asparagus, trimmed, cut into 1-inch pieces
  2 tablespoons sliced green onions (green part only)
1/4 cup shredded Parmesan cheese

> **COOK'S TIP**
>
> *Some suggestions for substitutions include strips of bell pepper, cubed eggplant, cauliflower, broccoli, or corn instead of yellow summer squash; snow peas, sugar snap peas, baby spinach, or bok choy leaves and stems instead of asparagus; and fresh dill, oregano, basil, marjoram, thyme, or lemon thyme instead of rosemary.*

1 In a large saucepan, bring 3 cups broth, potatoes, carrots, and pearl onions to a simmer over medium-high heat. Reduce the heat and simmer, covered, for 15 minutes, or until the potatoes and carrots are tender.

2 Stir in the zucchini, yellow squash, mushrooms, rosemary, salt, and pepper. Simmer, covered, for 3 to 4 minutes, or until both squashes are slightly tender.

3 In a small bowl, whisk together the remaining 1 cup broth and flour. Stir the broth mixture, asparagus, and green onions into the stew. Simmer, uncovered, for 2 to 3 minutes, or until the mixture has thickened and the asparagus is tender-crisp.

4 To serve, ladle into bowls. Top each serving with the Parmesan.

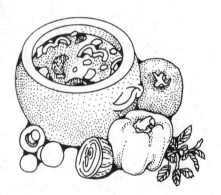

EXCHANGES

1 1/2 Starch
2 Vegetable
1/2 Fat

Calories 187
   Calories from Fat 36
Total Fat............................4 g
   Saturated Fat ....1.5 g
   Polyunsaturated Fat ....0.7 g
   Monounsaturated Fat .....1.0 g
Cholesterol ....9 mg
Sodium.........................469 mg
Total Carbohydrate........30 g
   Dietary Fiber ....4 g
   Sugars ....7 g
Protein ....10 g

Italian Lentil Soup

Leftovers of this lentil soup are even better than the just-prepared soup, for the flavors have had a chance to mingle.

Serves 5; 1 1/2 cups per serving

1 teaspoon olive oil
1/2 cup diced onion
8 ounces button mushrooms, sliced
2 medium garlic cloves, minced
4 cups low-fat, low-sodium chicken broth
14.5-ounce can no-salt-added tomatoes, undrained
1 cup dried lentils, sorted for stones and shriveled lentils and rinsed
1 teaspoon dried oregano, crumbled
1/4 teaspoon salt
1/4 teaspoon pepper
1 medium zucchini, diced
1 medium yellow summer squash, diced
1/2 cup shredded Parmesan cheese

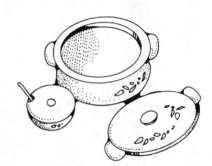

EXCHANGES

1 1/2 Starch
1 Lean Meat
2 Vegetable

Calories 239
  Calories from Fat 54
Total Fat..............................6 g
  Saturated Fat ....2.1 g
  Polyunsaturated Fat ....1.0 g
  Monounsaturated Fat .....2.0 g
Cholesterol ....11 mg
Sodium..........................318 mg
Total Carbohydrate.........32 g
  Dietary Fiber ....11 g
  Sugars ....9 g
Protein ....18 g

1. Heat a large saucepan or Dutch oven over medium-high heat. Pour in the oil and swirl to coat the bottom. Cook the onion for 2 to 3 minutes, or until tender, stirring occasionally.

2. Stir in the mushrooms and garlic. Cook for 2 to 3 minutes, or until the mushrooms are tender, stirring occasionally.

3. Stir in the broth, undrained tomatoes, lentils, oregano, salt, and pepper. Bring to a simmer, stirring occasionally. Cover the pan. Reduce the heat and simmer for 30 minutes, or until the lentils are almost tender (no stirring needed).

4. Stir in the zucchini and yellow squash. Cook, covered, for 15 minutes, or until the lentils and vegetables are tender.

5. To serve, ladle into bowls. Top each serving with 1 1/2 tablespoons Parmesan.

Salads

Mixed Green Salad with Peppery Citrus Dressing

Grapefruit zest and lemon zest give this salad its pizzazz.

Serves 5; 1 1/2 cups salad and 2 tablespoons dressing per serving

 6 cups mixed salad greens
 1 cup thinly sliced red onion
 1 cup snipped fresh cilantro

PEPPERY CITRUS DRESSING
 1/2 tablespoon grated grapefruit zest
 1/2 cup fresh grapefruit juice
 1 teaspoon grated lemon zest
 1 1/2 tablespoons fresh lemon juice
 1/2 tablespoon sugar
 1/2 tablespoon canola oil
 1 small fresh jalapeño pepper, seeds and ribs discarded, minced

1 Arrange the salad greens on a platter. Top with the onion and cilantro.

2 For the dressing, put the ingredients in a small jar with a tight-fitting lid. Shake vigorously to blend. Pour over the salad mixture. Serve immediately.

EXCHANGES

1/2 Fat
1/2 Carbohydrate

Calories	54
Calories from Fat	14
Total Fat	2 g
Saturated Fat	0.1 g
Polyunsaturated Fat	0.5 g
Monounsaturated Fat	0.8 g
Cholesterol	0 mg
Sodium	13 mg
Total Carbohydrate	9 g
Dietary Fiber	2 g
Sugars	7 g
Protein	1 g

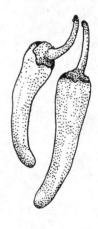

Salad Greens with Mixed-Herb Vinaigrette

Delicate baby salad greens and intensely flavored vinaigrette complement each other in this simple salad. The vinaigrette is also very good on thin slices of vine-ripened tomato.

Serves 5; about 2 cups greens and 2 heaping tablespoons dressing per serving

MIXED-HERB VINAIGRETTE
- 1/3 cup finely chopped fresh basil or 1 1/2 tablespoons dried basil, crumbled
- 1/4 cup dry white wine (regular or nonalcoholic)
- 2 tablespoons chopped fresh oregano or 2 teaspoons dried oregano, crumbled
- 2 tablespoons olive oil (extra virgin preferred)
- 1 teaspoon grated lemon zest
- 2 tablespoons fresh lemon juice
- 1/2 tablespoon cider vinegar
- 1/2 tablespoon Dijon mustard
- 1 medium garlic clove, minced
- 1/2 teaspoon salt
- 1/4 teaspoon pepper

SALAD
- 10 cups mixed salad greens (baby greens preferred)

1 Put the vinaigrette ingredients in a small jar with a tight-fitting lid. Shake vigorously until completely blended.

2 Just before serving, put the salad greens in a salad bowl. Shake the vinaigrette again. Pour it over the salad. Toss gently.

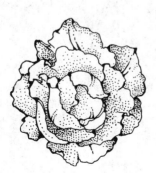

EXCHANGES

1 Vegetable
1 Fat

Calories	77
Calories from Fat	51
Total Fat	6 g
Saturated Fat	0.7 g
Polyunsaturated Fat	0.6 g
Monounsaturated Fat	4.0 g
Cholesterol	0 mg
Sodium	286 mg
Total Carbohydrate	4 g
Dietary Fiber	1 g
Sugars	3 g
Protein	1 g

Wedge Salad with Gorgonzola and Walnuts

Dijon mustard and garlic perk up a basic dressing for an iceberg wedge.

Serves 4; 1 lettuce wedge and 2 tablespoons dressing per serving

DRESSING
1/4 cup fat-free or low-fat plain yogurt
3 tablespoons fat-free milk
2 tablespoons fat-free or light mayonnaise dressing
1 teaspoon Dijon mustard
1/2 medium garlic clove, minced
1/4 teaspoon salt

SALAD
1 medium head of iceberg lettuce, cut into 4 wedges (about 3 ounces each)
1/2 cup finely chopped green onions (green and white parts)
1 ounce crumbled Gorgonzola cheese
1 tablespoon plus 1 teaspoon chopped walnuts, dry-roasted

1 In a small bowl, whisk together the dressing ingredients.

2 Place the lettuce wedges on a platter. Spoon the dressing over all. Sprinkle with the green onions, cheese, and walnuts.

EXCHANGES

1 Vegetable
1 Fat

Calories	71
Calories from Fat	32
Total Fat	4 g
Saturated Fat	1.3 g
Polyunsaturated Fat	1.0 g
Monounsaturated Fat	0.9 g
Cholesterol	6 mg
Sodium	355 mg
Total Carbohydrate	6 g
Dietary Fiber	2 g
Sugars	3 g
Protein	4 g

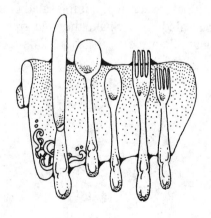

Tomato Salad with Creamy Horseradish Dressing

When tomatoes are at their best, this salad really shows them off.

Serves 4; 3 tomato slices and 2 tablespoons dressing per serving

CREAMY HORSERADISH DRESSING
1/3 cup fat-free or light sour cream
2 tablespoons fat-free or light mayonnaise dressing
1 teaspoon Dijon mustard
1 teaspoon prepared white horseradish
1/4 teaspoon salt
1/4 teaspoon pepper

SALAD
2 cups mixed salad greens
3 small tomatoes, each cut into 4 slices, or 12 ounces Italian plum tomatoes, sliced or quartered
Pepper to taste (optional)

1 In a small bowl, whisk together the dressing ingredients.

2 To serve, place the salad greens on a platter. Arrange the tomatoes on top. Spoon about 2 teaspoons dressing on each tomato slice. Sprinkle with additional pepper.

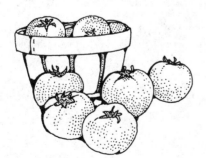

EXCHANGES

1/2 Carbohydrate

Calories	44
Calories from Fat	3
Total Fat	0 g
Saturated Fat	0 g
Polyunsaturated Fat	0.1 g
Monounsaturated Fat	0.1 g
Cholesterol	1 mg
Sodium	266 mg
Total Carbohydrate	9 g
Dietary Fiber	1 g
Sugars	5 g
Protein	2 g

Fanned Avocado Salad

This attractive salad is a real show-stopper!

Serves 6; 1/2 cup per serving

CITRUS DRESSING
  2 tablespoons fresh lime juice
  2 tablespoons fresh lemon juice
1/4 teaspoon salt
1/4 teaspoon black pepper
1/4 teaspoon red hot-pepper sauce

SALAD
16 medium spinach leaves
1/2 medium cucumber, peeled and sliced (about 4 ounces)
  1 medium tomato, sliced crosswise and halved (about 4 ounces)
  1 medium avocado, thinly sliced
1/2 cup snipped fresh cilantro
  1 ounce feta cheese, crumbled

1 In a small bowl, whisk together the dressing ingredients.

2 On a platter, decoratively arrange the spinach leaves, cucumber, tomato, and avocado slices like a fan or accordion. Spoon the dressing over all. Sprinkle with the cilantro and feta. Serve immediately so the spinach doesn't wilt and the flavors are more intense.

EXCHANGES

1 Vegetable
1 Fat

Calories 68
  Calories from Fat 45
Total Fat...........................5 g
  Saturated Fat ....1.3 g
  Polyunsaturated Fat ....0.6 g
  Monounsaturated Fat .....2.6 g
Cholesterol ....4 mg
Sodium..........................179 mg
Total Carbohydrate...........5 g
  Dietary Fiber ....2 g
  Sugars ....2 g
Protein ....2 g

Chopped Veggie Salad with Feta

When you want a change from tossed green salad, try this easy alternative.

Serves 4; 3/4 cup per serving

1/2 14-ounce can quartered artichoke hearts, rinsed, drained, and coarsely chopped
  4 ounces button mushrooms, chopped (about 1/4-inch cubes)
  1 small tomato, seeded and chopped
1/4 cup finely chopped green onions (green and white parts)
1/4 cup snipped fresh parsley
1/2 tablespoon dried basil, crumbled
3/4 teaspoon dried oregano, crumbled
1/2 ounce feta cheese with sun-dried tomatoes and basil, crumbled

In a medium bowl, toss together all the ingredients except the feta. Add the feta and toss gently. This salad is best if served within 1 hour of preparation.

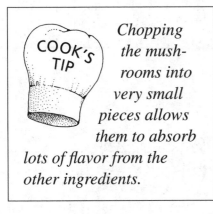

COOK'S TIP

Chopping the mushrooms into very small pieces allows them to absorb lots of flavor from the other ingredients.

EXCHANGES

1 Vegetable

Calories 39
  Calories from Fat 11
Total Fat............................1 g
  Saturated Fat ....0.6 g
  Polyunsaturated Fat ....0.2 g
  Monounsaturated Fat .....0.2 g
Cholesterol ....2 mg
Sodium..........................123 mg
Total Carbohydrate...........6 g
  Dietary Fiber ....1 g
  Sugars ....2 g
Protein ....2 g

Crunchy Asian Snow Pea Salad

This kaleidoscope-colored salad is just right with Asian entrées or as a change from coleslaw at picnics and barbecues. (See photo insert.)

Serves 4; 1/2 cup per serving

SALAD
1/2 8-ounce can sliced water chestnuts, rinsed, drained, and halved
1/2 cup finely chopped red onion
1/2 medium yellow bell pepper, finely chopped
3 ounces fresh snow peas (do not use frozen), trimmed, cut diagonally into 1/2-inch pieces
2 tablespoons snipped fresh cilantro

DRESSING
2 tablespoons fresh lemon juice
1/2 tablespoon sugar
1/2 tablespoon canola oil
1 teaspoon grated peeled gingerroot

1 In a medium bowl, stir together the salad ingredients.

2 Put the dressing ingredients in a jar with a tight-fitting lid. Shake vigorously to blend well. Pour over the salad. Toss gently.

EXCHANGES

1 Vegetable
1/2 Fat

Calories	50
Calories from Fat	16
Total Fat	2 g
Saturated Fat	0.1 g
Polyunsaturated Fat	0.5 g
Monounsaturated Fat	1.0 g
Cholesterol	0 mg
Sodium	6 mg
Total Carbohydrate	8 g
Dietary Fiber	1 g
Sugars	5 g
Protein	1 g

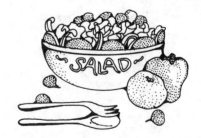

Fiesta Slaw

Although this sweet and tangy coleslaw is good with almost any entrée, it is especially well suited to Mexican food. Try it with Fabulous Fajitas (page 108).

Serves 5; 1/2 cup per serving

  2 cups packaged shredded coleslaw mix
1/2 cup diced yellow summer squash
1/2 poblano pepper, seeds and ribs discarded, chopped
1/4 medium red bell pepper, chopped
1/4 cup snipped fresh cilantro
1 1/2 tablespoons fat-free or light mayonnaise dressing
1/2 tablespoon fresh lime juice
1/2 tablespoon sugar (2 teaspoons if using light mayonnaise dressing)
1/8 teaspoon salt

In a large bowl, toss all the ingredients to coat. Serve immediately for peak flavor (the flavor begins to break down if the salad is chilled).

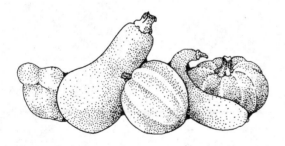

EXCHANGES

1 Vegetable

Calories	22
Calories from Fat	1
Total Fat	0 g
Saturated Fat	0 g
Polyunsaturated Fat	0.1 g
Monounsaturated Fat	0 g
Cholesterol	0 mg
Sodium	100 mg
Total Carbohydrate	5 g
Dietary Fiber	1 g
Sugars	3 g
Protein	1 g

Italian Salsa Salad

Bigger chunks of veggies turn Italian-inspired salsa into a sensational salad.

Serves 6; 1/2 cup per serving

10 ounces grape tomatoes or cherry tomatoes, halved (about 2 cups)
1/2 medium green bell pepper, chopped
1/2 cup chopped red onion
1/2 cup snipped fresh parsley
3 tablespoons capers, rinsed and drained
2 tablespoons cider vinegar
1 tablespoon olive oil (extra virgin preferred)
2 teaspoons dried basil, crumbled
1 teaspoon dried oregano, crumbled
1/8 teaspoon crushed red pepper flakes
1/4 teaspoon salt

In a medium bowl, gently toss all the ingredients. Let stand for 10 minutes before serving.

EXCHANGES

1 Vegetable
1/2 Fat

Calories 43
Calories from Fat 23
Total Fat.............................3 g
Saturated Fat ....0.3 g
Polyunsaturated Fat ....0.3 g
Monounsaturated Fat .....1.7 g
Cholesterol ....0 mg
Sodium...........................232 mg
Total Carbohydrate...........5 g
Dietary Fiber ....2 g
Sugars ....3 g
Protein ....1 g

COOK'S TIP

A variety of cherry tomato, the grape tomato is sweet and less watery than its relative. That means it won't break down the intensity of other ingredients.

Farmer's Market Veggie Salad

If you like your salad fresh, crisp, and colorful, this will become a favorite.

Serves 4; 1/2 cup per serving

    1/2 medium yellow bell pepper, thinly sliced
      1 small carrot, thinly sliced
      1 ounce snow peas, trimmed
    1/4 cup thinly sliced red onion
  2 1/4 teaspoons canola oil
    1/2 tablespoon cider vinegar
    1/2 tablespoon sugar
    1/8 teaspoon salt
         Dash of red hot-pepper sauce, or to taste

In a large bowl, toss together all the ingredients. Serve immediately for peak flavor.

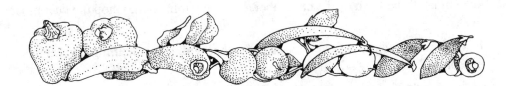

EXCHANGES

1 Vegetable
1/2 Fat

Calories	46
Calories from Fat	24
Total Fat	3 g
Saturated Fat	0.2 g
Polyunsaturated Fat	0.8 g
Monounsaturated Fat	1.5 g
Cholesterol	0 mg
Sodium	81 mg
Total Carbohydrate	6 g
Dietary Fiber	1 g
Sugars	4 g
Protein	1 g

Black-Bean Cucumber Boats

With their visual appeal, these cucumber boats are a great choice when it's your turn to bring the salad.

Serves 4; 1 stuffed cucumber half per serving

- 2 large cucumbers, cut in half lengthwise
- 1/2 15-ounce can no-salt-added black beans, rinsed and drained
- 1 medium Anaheim pepper, seeds and ribs discarded, finely chopped
- 1/3 cup finely chopped red onion
- 1/4 cup snipped fresh cilantro
- 2 tablespoons cider vinegar
- 2 tablespoons fresh lime juice
- 1/4 teaspoon salt
- 1 tablespoon olive oil (extra virgin preferred)

1 Using a spoon, remove and discard the cucumber seeds. Carefully scoop out and keep most of the flesh of the cucumber, leaving a thin shell. Chop the cucumber flesh.

2 In a medium bowl, toss the chopped cucumber with the remaining ingredients except the oil. Gently stir in the oil.

3 To serve, spoon the bean mixture into each cucumber half.

EXCHANGES

1/2 Starch
1 Vegetable
1 Fat

Calories 103
  Calories from Fat 33
Total Fat...........................4 g
  Saturated Fat ....0.5 g
  Polyunsaturated Fat ....0.5 g
  Monounsaturated Fat .....2.5 g
Cholesterol ....0 mg
Sodium..........................151 mg
Total Carbohydrate........15 g
  Dietary Fiber ....3 g
  Sugars ....5 g
Protein ....4 g

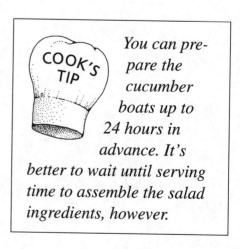

COOK'S TIP

You can prepare the cucumber boats up to 24 hours in advance. It's better to wait until serving time to assemble the salad ingredients, however.

Confetti Garden Salad

There's just something about a cold, creamy salad that sets off a meal.

Serves 6; 1/2 cup per serving

DRESSING
3 tablespoons fat-free or light mayonnaise dressing
1/2 tablespoon dried dill weed, crumbled
1/2 tablespoon Dijon mustard
1/2 teaspoon sugar
1/4 teaspoon salt

SALAD
1 large red bell pepper, chopped
1 medium cucumber, peeled, seeded, and chopped
1 medium rib of celery, chopped
1/2 cup frozen green peas
1/2 cup frozen whole-kernel corn

1 In a medium bowl, whisk together the dressing ingredients.

2 Add the remaining ingredients. Using a rubber scraper so you can incorporate all the dressing, stir together gently.

3 Let stand for 15 minutes to absorb flavors. Serve within another 15 minutes for the best texture and flavor (the dressing begins to break down if it stands too long).

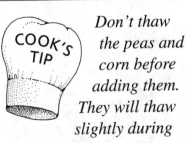

COOK'S TIP

Don't thaw the peas and corn before adding them. They will thaw slightly during the standing time, giving the dish a fresh taste and good texture.

EXCHANGES

1/2 Carbohydrate

Calories	44
Calories from Fat	2
Total Fat	0 g
Saturated Fat	0 g
Polyunsaturated Fat	0.1 g
Monounsaturated Fat	0 g
Cholesterol	0 mg
Sodium	199 mg
Total Carbohydrate	9 g
Dietary Fiber	2 g
Sugars	3 g
Protein	2 g

Chunky Potato Salad

Flecks of red and green brighten up this zippy potato salad. Double the recipe if you have a larger gathering.

Serves 4; 1/2 cup per serving

    8 ounces red potatoes, cut into 1/2-inch cubes
  1/2 medium green bell pepper, finely chopped
  1/2 medium rib of celery, finely chopped
  1/4 cup finely chopped red onion
1 1/2 tablespoons fat-free or light mayonnaise dressing
    1 tablespoon fat-free or light sour cream
2 1/4 teaspoons cider vinegar
    1 teaspoon prepared mustard
  1/4 teaspoon salt

1 Set a steamer basket in a small amount of simmering water in a medium saucepan. Put the potatoes in the basket. Cook, covered, for 8 to 10 minutes, or until tender.

2 Transfer to a colander and run under cold water until completely cooled. Shake off the excess liquid.

3 Meanwhile, in a medium bowl, stir together the remaining ingredients.

4 Stir the potatoes into the bell pepper mixture. Cover with plastic wrap and refrigerate for 30 minutes.

EXCHANGES

1 Starch

Calories	65
Calories from Fat	1
Total Fat	0 g
Saturated Fat	0 g
Polyunsaturated Fat	0.1 g
Monounsaturated Fat	0 g
Cholesterol	0 mg
Sodium	210 mg
Total Carbohydrate	15 g
Dietary Fiber	2 g
Sugars	3 g
Protein	2 g

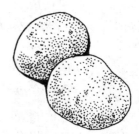

Cantaloupe Wedges with Ginger-Citrus Sauce

This versatile dish is great for breakfast, brunch, lunch, or dinner.

Serves 4; 2 cantaloupe wedges, 2 tablespoons blueberries, and 2 tablespoons sauce per serving

GINGER-CITRUS SAUCE
1/4 cup frozen orange juice concentrate
1 teaspoon grated lemon zest
2 tablespoons fresh lemon juice
1 1/2 tablespoons honey
1 teaspoon grated peeled gingerroot

FRUIT
1-pound cantaloupe, peeled, seeded, and cut into 8 wedges or diced
1/2 cup blueberries

1. In a small bowl, whisk together the sauce ingredients.

2. Arrange the cantaloupe on a platter, sprinkle with the blueberries, and spoon the sauce over the fruit. Serve immediately for peak flavor.

EXCHANGES

1 1/2 Fruit

Calories	85
Calories from Fat	2
Total Fat	0 g
Saturated Fat	0 g
Polyunsaturated Fat	0 g
Monounsaturated Fat	0 g
Cholesterol	0 mg
Sodium	9 mg
Total Carbohydrate	21 g
Dietary Fiber	1 g
Sugars	19 g
Protein	1 g

Caribbean Fruit Salad Platter

Whether you're entertaining overnighters, having a patio party, or going to a family reunion, this will be a refreshing, brilliantly colored hit. If you want fewer servings, it's easy to reduce the amounts.

Serves 12; 1/2 cup per serving

1/2 cup sweetened flaked coconut
2 cups quartered strawberries
1 medium banana, sliced diagonally
1 medium mango, cubed
2 kiwifruit, peeled and cut into wedges
1 teaspoon grated orange zest
Juice of 1 medium orange
1 teaspoon grated lemon zest
1 tablespoon fresh lemon juice
1/2 tablespoon sugar

1 Heat a large nonstick skillet over medium-high heat. Lightly brown the coconut for 1 to 2 minutes, stirring constantly. Remove from the heat.

2 Arrange the strawberries, banana, mango, and kiwifruit on a platter.

3 In a small bowl, whisk together the remaining ingredients. Pour over the fruit. Sprinkle with the coconut.

EXCHANGES

1 Fruit

Calories	60
Calories from Fat	12
Total Fat	1 g
Saturated Fat	1.0 g
Polyunsaturated Fat	0 g
Monounsaturated Fat	0 g
Cholesterol	0 mg
Sodium	10 mg
Total Carbohydrate	13 g
Dietary Fiber	2 g
Sugars	10 g
Protein	1 g

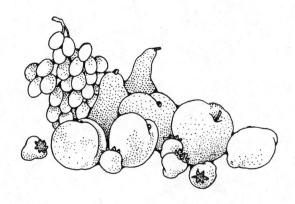

Tropical Lemon Gelatin

Although children love this colorful salad, it's dressed up enough to appeal to adults as well.

Serves 6; 1 wedge and about 1/3 cup fruit per serving

    0.3-ounce package sugar-free lemon gelatin (4-serving size)
1 cup boiling water
1/2 cup cold water
1 tablespoon fresh lemon juice

TOPPING
1 teaspoon grated lemon zest
1 cup fat-free or low-fat vanilla yogurt
1 kiwifruit, peeled and sliced
1/2 cup diced mango
1 cup quartered strawberries

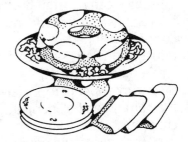

1 Put the gelatin in a 9-inch glass pie pan or 8- or 9-inch square glass baking dish. Pour in the boiling water. Stir until the gelatin is completely dissolved.

2 Stir in the cold water and lemon juice. Cover with plastic wrap. Refrigerate until firm, about 4 hours.

3 For the topping, stir the lemon zest into the yogurt. Spoon the yogurt evenly over the gelatin mixture. Arrange the fruit decoratively on the yogurt. Cut into wedges or squares. Serve within 2 hours of adding topping for best results.

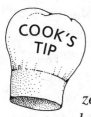

COOK'S TIP

It's easier to remove the zest of citrus fruit before squeezing out the juice. A rasp zester works well. Just be careful and don't grate the bitter white pith just below the peel.

EXCHANGES

1 Fruit

Calories	55
Calories from Fat	2
Total Fat	0 g
Saturated Fat	0 g
Polyunsaturated Fat	0 g
Monounsaturated Fat	0 g
Cholesterol	1 mg
Sodium	63 mg
Total Carbohydrate	11 g
Dietary Fiber	1 g
Sugars	8 g
Protein	3 g

Chicken Antipasto Salad

When you want to use up some leftover chicken, here's a filling salad to try.

Serves 4; heaping 1 1/2 cups per serving

- 3 ounces dried whole-wheat rotini
  14-ounce can quartered artichoke hearts, rinsed, drained, and coarsely chopped
- 8 ounces boneless, skinless cooked chicken breasts, diced
- 14 slices turkey pepperoni, halved
- 1 medium green bell pepper, finely chopped
- 1/2 cup thinly sliced red onion

- 1/2 cup chopped roasted red bell peppers, rinsed and drained if bottled
- 1/2 tablespoon dried basil, crumbled
- 1 tablespoon cider vinegar
- 1 tablespoon olive oil (extra virgin preferred)
- 1 1/2 ounces feta cheese with sun-dried tomato and basil, crumbled

1 Cook the pasta using the package directions, omitting the salt and oil. Drain in a colander. Run under cold water until completely cooled. Drain well.

2 Meanwhile, in a large bowl, stir together the artichokes, chicken, pepperoni, green bell pepper, onion, red bell pepper, and basil.

3 Add the pasta, vinegar, and oil to the artichoke mixture and toss gently. Add the feta and toss gently. Serve immediately for peak flavors.

EXCHANGES

1 Starch
3 Lean Meat
2 Vegetable

Calories	297
Calories from Fat	89
Total Fat	10 g
Saturated Fat	3.0 g
Polyunsaturated Fat	1.3 g
Monounsaturated Fat	4.0 g
Cholesterol	64 mg
Sodium	495 mg
Total Carbohydrate	26 g
Dietary Fiber	3 g
Sugars	5 g
Protein	26 g

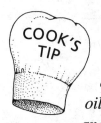

COOK'S TIP

To make this salad ahead, stir together all the ingredients except the vinegar, oil, and feta. Cover and refrigerate until needed. At serving time, add the vinegar and oil and toss gently. Add the feta and toss gently.

Cranberry-Pecan Turkey Salad

Leftovers from the Roast Turkey with Orange-Spice Rub (page 97) are especially good in this so-simple salad.

Serves 4; heaping 3/4 cup turkey mixture and 1/2 medium apple per serving

1/4 cup fat-free or low-fat vanilla yogurt
  2 tablespoons fat-free or light mayonnaise dressing
 12 ounces boneless, skinless cooked turkey breast, diced (about 2 1/2 cups)
1/2 cup dried cranberries
  1 medium rib of celery, sliced
1/4 cup finely chopped red onion
  1 ounce pecan chips, dry-roasted
  2 medium apples, sliced

1 In a medium bowl, stir together the yogurt and mayonnaise.

2 Stir in the turkey.

3 Stir in the remaining ingredients except the apple slices.

4 Fan the apple slices in a half-circle on each of four plates. Spoon the turkey mixture beside the apple slices.

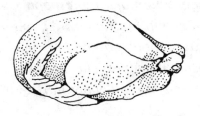

EXCHANGES

3 Very Lean Meat
2 Fruit
1 Fat

Calories 277
  Calories from Fat 59
Total Fat ....7 g
  Saturated Fat ....0.8 g
  Polyunsaturated Fat ....1.9 g
  Monounsaturated Fat .....3.1 g
Cholesterol ....69 mg
Sodium ....115 mg
Total Carbohydrate ....28 g
  Dietary Fiber ....4 g
  Sugars ....23 g
Protein ....27 g

Lemony Shrimp Salad

A triple dose of lemon—zest, juice, and slices—complements a triple dose of spicy seasonings—Creole seasoning, black pepper, and red hot-pepper sauce.

Serves 4; 3/4 cup shrimp mixture and 1 cup salad greens per serving

```
  6 cups water
  1 pound peeled raw medium shrimp
  2 large hard-cooked eggs
1/2 cup finely chopped green onions (green and white parts)
1/2 cup finely chopped celery
1/4 cup snipped fresh parsley
  1 teaspoon grated lemon zest
1/4 cup fresh lemon juice
  2 tablespoons fat-free or light sour cream
  2 tablespoons fat-free or light mayonnaise dressing
1/2 teaspoon Creole or Cajun seasoning
1/4 teaspoon salt
1/4 teaspoon black pepper
1/8 teaspoon red hot-pepper sauce
  4 cups mixed salad greens
  2 lemons, quartered
```

COOK'S TIP

We called for bottled Creole or Cajun seasoning in this recipe, but many of these blends are high in sodium. It's very easy to make your own salt-free mixture. Simply stir together a combination of 1 tablespoon each of chili powder, ground cumin, garlic powder, onion powder, and paprika, plus 2 teaspoons ground oregano, 2 teaspoons ground thyme, and 1/2 teaspoon pepper. The mixture will last for up to six months if you keep it at room temperature in a tightly covered container.

1   In a large saucepan, bring the water to a boil over high heat. Boil the shrimp for 3 minutes, or until pink on the outside and opaque in the center. Drain in a colander. Run cold water over the shrimp to cool them quickly. Drain well on paper towels.

2   Meanwhile, cut each egg in half. Discard 2 yolk halves. Chop the remaining 2 yolk halves and all the whites.

3   In a medium bowl, stir together the remaining ingredients except the salad greens and lemon. Add the shrimp and toss gently. Add the eggs and toss gently.

4   To serve, place 1 cup salad greens on each plate. Top each serving with a heaping 3/4 cup shrimp mixture. Place 2 lemon wedges on each plate to squeeze over the salad.

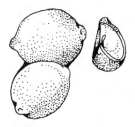

EXCHANGES

3 Very Lean Meat
1/2 Carbohydrate

Calories 147
   Calories from Fat 22
Total Fat...........................2 g
   Saturated Fat ....0.8 g
   Polyunsaturated Fat ....0.6 g
   Monounsaturated Fat .....0.7 g
Cholesterol ....228 mg
Sodium.........................498 mg
Total Carbohydrate..........8 g
   Dietary Fiber ....1 g
   Sugars ....4 g
Protein ....23 g

Seafood

Tilapia with Dill and Paprika

Here's a simple recipe to try if you are a bit hesitant to cook fish. The preparation is easy, and the seasonings are light—sure to please almost everyone.

Serves 4; 3 ounces fish per serving

Vegetable oil spray (olive oil spray preferred)
4 tilapia or other thin, mild fish fillets (about 4 ounces each)
1 teaspoon dried dill weed, crumbled
3/4 teaspoon paprika
1/4 teaspoon salt
1/4 teaspoon pepper
2 medium lemons, quartered

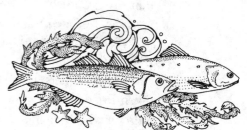

1 Preheat the oven to 350°F.

2 Lightly spray a nonstick baking sheet with vegetable oil spray. Rinse the fish and pat dry with paper towels. Place the fish on the baking sheet.

3 In a small bowl, stir together the dill weed, paprika, salt, and pepper. Sprinkle over the fish. Lightly spray the fish with vegetable oil spray.

4 Bake for 10 to 12 minutes, or until the fish flakes easily when tested with a fork.

5 To serve, place the fish on plates. Place 2 lemon quarters on each plate to squeeze over the fish.

EXCHANGES

3 Very Lean Meat

Calories	118
Calories from Fat	23
Total Fat	3 g
Saturated Fat	1.0 g
Polyunsaturated Fat	0.7 g
Monounsaturated Fat	0.7 g
Cholesterol	76 mg
Sodium	181 mg
Total Carbohydrate	2 g
Dietary Fiber	0 g
Sugars	1 g
Protein	23 g

Pan-Fried Catfish with Fresh Veggie Relish

Crisp, flavor-packed ingredients give this vegetable relish that extra-fresh taste. You can serve it on the spicy fish or as an unusual side dish.

Serves 4; 3 ounces fish and about 1/4 cup relish per serving

RELISH
1 medium red bell pepper, very finely chopped
1 cup very finely chopped carrots
2 tablespoons very finely chopped red onion
2 tablespoons fresh lemon juice
1/2 tablespoon sugar
3/4 teaspoon grated peeled gingerroot

CATFISH
1/2 teaspoon chili powder
1/2 teaspoon dried oregano, crumbled
1/4 teaspoon salt
1/4 teaspoon black pepper
4 catfish fillets (about 4 ounces each)
2 teaspoons canola oil

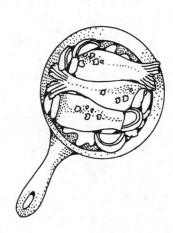

1 In a medium bowl, stir together all the relish ingredients. Set aside.

2 In a small bowl, stir together the chili powder, oregano, salt, and black pepper. Rinse the fish and pat dry with paper towels. Rub the chili powder mixture evenly over the fish.

3 Heat a 12-inch nonstick skillet over medium-high heat. Add the oil and swirl to coat the bottom. When the oil is hot, cook the fish for 3 minutes on each side, or until it flakes easily when tested with a fork.

4 To serve, place the fish on plates. Serve with the relish spooned on top or to the side.

EXCHANGES

3 Lean Meat
1 Vegetable

Calories	210
Calories from Fat	88
Total Fat	10 g
Saturated Fat	2.6 g
Polyunsaturated Fat	2.0 g
Monounsaturated Fat	5.0 g
Cholesterol	61 mg
Sodium	219 mg
Total Carbohydrate	8 g
Dietary Fiber	2 g
Sugars	5 g
Protein	21 g

Cornmeal-Coated Baked Catfish with Italian Tomato Sauce

Catfish with a hint of orange in its cornmeal coating partners well with oregano-infused tomato sauce.

Serves 4; 3 ounces fish and 2 tablespoons sauce per serving

TOMATO SAUCE
- 1 teaspoon olive oil
- 1 small onion, chopped
- 2 tablespoons grated carrot
- 1 medium garlic clove, minced
- 8-ounce can no-salt-added tomato sauce
- 2 tablespoons snipped fresh Italian (flat-leaf) parsley
- 1/2 teaspoon dried oregano, crumbled
- 1/4 teaspoon crushed red pepper flakes

CATFISH
- 1/3 cup fat-free or low-fat buttermilk
- 1 tablespoon fresh orange juice
- 1 teaspoon grated orange zest
- 1/2 cup yellow cornmeal
- 1 medium Anaheim pepper, seeded and ribs discarded, finely chopped
- 1/4 teaspoon salt
- Vegetable oil spray
- 4 catfish fillets (about 4 ounces each)

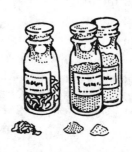

1 For the sauce, heat a medium nonstick skillet over medium heat. Pour in the oil and swirl to coat the bottom. Cook the onion, carrot, and garlic for 2 to 3 minutes, or until the onion is tender, stirring occasionally.

2 Stir in the remaining sauce ingredients. Increase the heat to medium high and bring to a boil. Reduce the heat and simmer, partially covered, for 20 minutes. Meanwhile, preheat the oven to 450°F.

3 In a shallow dish or pie pan, whisk together the buttermilk and orange juice.

4 In another shallow dish or pie pan, stir together the orange zest, cornmeal, Anaheim pepper, and salt. Place the dishes side by side.

5 Lightly spray an 11 × 7 × 2-inch baking pan with vegetable oil spray. Set beside the cornmeal mixture.

6 Rinse the fish and pat dry with paper towels. Dip the fish into the buttermilk mixture, turning to coat. Roll the fish in the cornmeal mixture, shaking off any excess. Place the fish in a single layer in the baking pan. Lightly spray the top of the fish with vegetable oil spray.

7 Bake, uncovered, for 12 to 15 minutes, or until the top coating is slightly crisp and the fish flakes easily when tested with a fork.

8 To serve, place the fish on plates. Pour about 2 tablespoons sauce over each serving.

EXCHANGES

1/2 Starch
3 Lean Meat
2 Vegetable

Calories	257
Calories from Fat	88
Total Fat	10 g
Saturated Fat	2.1 g
Polyunsaturated Fat	1.7 g
Monounsaturated Fat	5.2 g
Cholesterol	66 mg
Sodium	234 mg
Total Carbohydrate	19 g
Dietary Fiber	3 g
Sugars	7 g
Protein	22 g

Baked Fish Sticks with a Kick

These fish sticks are all grown up, with tang from buttermilk, yogurt, and lemon juice, plus zip from horseradish, Dijon mustard, and pepper.

Serves 4; 3 ounces fish per serving

1/3 cup finely crushed reduced-sodium five-grain crispbread or whole-wheat crackers
1/4 cup yellow cornmeal
1/4 cup fat-free or low-fat buttermilk
1/4 cup fat-free or low-fat plain yogurt
2 tablespoons fresh lemon juice

1 tablespoon prepared white horseradish
1 teaspoon Dijon mustard
1/2 teaspoon dried thyme, crumbled
1/4 teaspoon pepper
Vegetable oil spray
1 pound cod, orange roughy, or other firm white fish fillets

1 Preheat the oven to 475°F.

2 In a shallow dish or pie pan, stir together the crispbread crumbs and cornmeal.

3 In another shallow dish or pie pan, whisk together the remaining ingredients except the fish. Place the dishes side by side.

4 Lightly spray a baking sheet with vegetable oil spray. Set beside the buttermilk mixture.

5 Rinse the fish and pat dry with paper towels. Cut the fish crosswise into 3/4-inch strips. Dip the fish into the buttermilk mixture, turning to coat. Roll the fish in the crispbread mixture, shaking off any excess. Place the fish sticks in a single layer on the baking sheet. Lightly spray the top of the fish with vegetable oil spray.

6 Bake for 12 to 15 minutes, or until the fish flakes easily when tested with a fork and the top coating is crisp and golden.

EXCHANGES

1 Starch
3 Very Lean Meat

Calories 160
Calories from Fat 11
Total Fat.............................1 g
Saturated Fat ....0.3 g
Polyunsaturated Fat ....0.4 g
Monounsaturated Fat .....0.2 g
Cholesterol ....49 mg
Sodium...........................154 mg
Total Carbohydrate.........14 g
Dietary Fiber ....2 g
Sugars ....2 g
Protein ....23 g

COOK'S TIP

It is easier to cut the fish into sticks when it is very cold or slightly frozen.

Baked Fish Fillets with Thyme-Dijon Topping

This spicy Louisiana favorite commands center stage. Add hot, fluffy rice and a steamed veggie to round out the meal.

Serves 4; 3 ounces fish and 1 tablespoon topping per serving

Vegetable oil spray
4 grouper or other mild fish fillets (about 4 ounces each)
3 tablespoons light tub margarine
2 tablespoons finely snipped fresh parsley
1 teaspoon Dijon mustard
1/4 teaspoon dried thyme, crumbled
1/4 teaspoon red hot-pepper sauce
1/8 teaspoon salt

1 Preheat the oven to 350°F. Lightly spray a nonstick baking sheet with vegetable oil spray. Rinse the fish and pat dry with paper towels. Place the fish on the baking sheet.

2 Bake for 18 to 20 minutes, or until the fish flakes easily when tested with a fork.

3 Meanwhile, in a small bowl, stir together the remaining ingredients.

4 To serve, place the fish on a platter. Spoon the margarine mixture over the fish. Spread to coat the surface.

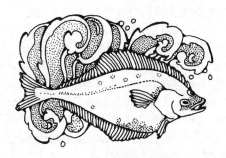

EXCHANGES

3 Very Lean Meat
1/2 Fat

Calories 137
Calories from Fat 41
Total Fat .... 5 g
Saturated Fat .... 0.3 g
Polyunsaturated Fat .... 1.1 g
Monounsaturated Fat ..... 2.1 g
Cholesterol .... 42 mg
Sodium .... 223 mg
Total Carbohydrate .... 0 g
Dietary Fiber .... 0 g
Sugars .... 0 g
Protein .... 22 g

Oven-Fried Haddock Sandwich

Serve these fish sandwiches with baked sweet-potato fries and coleslaw. Pop the potatoes in the oven at the same time as the haddock.

Serves 4; 1 sandwich per serving

HADDOCK
1/3 cup fat-free evaporated milk
1 teaspoon grated lemon zest
2 tablespoons fresh lemon juice
1 tablespoon prepared white horseradish
1/3 cup finely crushed reduced-sodium five-grain crispbread or whole-wheat crackers
1/4 cup yellow cornmeal
1/4 teaspoon crushed red pepper flakes
Vegetable oil spray
1 pound haddock or other mild fish fillets, such as cod or flounder

TARTAR SAUCE
2 tablespoons fat-free or light mayonnaise dressing
1 teaspoon minced red onion
1 teaspoon minced fresh Italian (flat-leaf) parsley
1 teaspoon minced sweet pickle or cornichon

SANDWICHES
4 whole-wheat sandwich rolls or buns
4 medium-large lettuce leaves, any variety
8 slices tomato

1 Preheat the oven to 450°F.

2 In a shallow glass bowl or pie pan, stir together the evaporated milk, lemon zest, lemon juice, and horseradish.

3 In another shallow bowl or pie pan, stir together the cracker crumbs, cornmeal, and red pepper flakes. Place the bowls side by side.

4 Lightly spray a baking pan or baking sheet with vegetable oil spray. Set beside the cracker crumb mixture.

5 Rinse the fish and pat dry with paper towels. Dip the fish into the milk mixture, turning to coat. Roll the fish in the cracker crumb mixture, shaking off any excess. Place the fish in the baking pan. Lightly spray the top of the fish with vegetable oil spray.

6 Bake for 12 to 14 minutes, or until the fish flakes easily when tested with a fork.

7 Meanwhile, in a small bowl, stir together the tartar sauce ingredients.

8 To assemble, spread 1 teaspoon tartar sauce on the top piece of each roll. Place the fish, lettuce, and 2 tomato slices on the bottom piece of each roll. Put the top on each sandwich.

EXCHANGES

2 1/2 Starch
3 Very Lean Meat

Calories	296
Calories from Fat	35
Total Fat	4 g
Saturated Fat	0.8 g
Polyunsaturated Fat	0.9 g
Monounsaturated Fat	1.4 g
Cholesterol	65 mg
Sodium	393 mg
Total Carbohydrate	37 g
Dietary Fiber	4 g
Sugars	7 g
Protein	29 g

Salmon with Mango and Peach Salsa

Packed with the natural sweetness of mango and peaches, the salsa in this dish gets its kick from hot peppers, cumin, and coriander. (See photo insert.)

Serves 4; 3 ounces fish and 2 tablespoons salsa per serving

Vegetable oil spray

SALSA
1 medium mango, chopped
1 cup chopped fresh peeled peaches or 8-ounce can light peaches in extra-light syrup, drained and chopped
3 tablespoons chopped red onion
1 small fresh jalapeño pepper, seeds and ribs discarded, chopped, or 1/2 teaspoon bottled pickled jalapeño juice

1/4 cup snipped fresh cilantro or fresh Italian (flat-leaf) parsley
1 teaspoon grated lime zest
2 tablespoons fresh lime juice
1/4 teaspoon ground cumin

SALMON
4 salmon fillets with skin (5 to 6 ounces each)
1/4 teaspoon salt
1/4 teaspoon pepper (white preferred)

1. Lightly spray a grill rack with vegetable oil spray. Preheat the grill to medium-high.

2. In a medium bowl, stir together the salsa ingredients.

3. Rinse the fish and pat dry with paper towels. Season with the salt and pepper.

4. Grill the salmon with the skin side up for 4 minutes, or until browned. Using a spatula, turn the fish over. Grill for 3 to 4 minutes, or until the fish flakes easily when tested with a fork.

5. To serve, place the fish with the skin side down on plates. Spoon the salsa on top or to the side of the fish.

EXCHANGES

4 Lean Meat
1 Fruit

Calories	304
Calories from Fat	112
Total Fat	12 g
Saturated Fat	2.2 g
Polyunsaturated Fat	2.8 g
Monounsaturated Fat	6.0 g
Cholesterol	96 mg
Sodium	222 mg
Total Carbohydrate	17 g
Dietary Fiber	2 g
Sugars	13 g
Protein	31 g

Salmon Tacos

Soft tortillas envelop a filling of grilled salmon, coleslaw, and tomato. One bite and you'll shout ¡Olé!

Serves 4; 1 taco per serving

SLAW

1/4	cup fat-free or low-fat plain yogurt
1	teaspoon grated lime zest
1/4	teaspoon chili powder
1 1/2	cups shredded cabbage or green-leaf lettuce
1/4	medium red or green bell pepper, chopped
2	tablespoons finely chopped red onion
1/2	tablespoon grated radish
1	teaspoon minced fresh jalapeño pepper, seeds and ribs discarded

TACOS

12	ounces skinless salmon or cod fillets, cut into 4 pieces
	Vegetable oil spray
4	6-inch whole-wheat or spinach tortillas
1/2	cup chopped tomato
2	tablespoons fat-free or light sour cream
2	teaspoons fresh lime juice
2	teaspoons snipped fresh cilantro or Italian (flat-leaf) parsley

1 For the slaw, in a small bowl, stir together the yogurt, lime zest, and chili powder.

2 In a medium bowl, stir together the remaining slaw ingredients. Add the yogurt mixture and toss to coat.

3 Rinse the fish and pat dry with paper towels. Heat a ridged grill pan over medium-high heat. Remove from the heat and lightly spray with vegetable oil spray (being careful not to spray near a gas flame).

4 Cook the fish for 8 to 9 minutes, turning once, or until the fish flakes easily when tested with a fork. Or lightly spray an outdoor grill rack and heat on medium high. Grill the fish as directed. Place on a plate. Cover with aluminum foil to keep warm.

5 Heat a small nonstick skillet over medium heat. Warm a tortilla for 30 seconds. Turn over and warm for 20 to 30 seconds, or until pliable. Put on a small plate and cover with a barely damp dish towel. Repeat with the remaining tortillas. Or stack the tortillas and wrap them in a slightly damp paper towel. Microwave for 12 to 15 seconds on 100 percent power (high).

6 To assemble, spoon the slaw on the upper third of each tortilla. Break the salmon into chunks. Put the salmon on the slaw. Sprinkle with the tomato. Fold in both sides of each tortilla. Roll up the tortilla from the filling end to the bottom.

7 In a small bowl, stir together the remaining ingredients. Spoon the mixture over each taco.

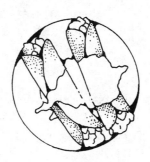

EXCHANGES

1 Starch
3 Lean Meat
1 Vegetable

Calories 265
   Calories from Fat 88
Total Fat ....10 g
   Saturated Fat ....1.6 g
   Polyunsaturated Fat ....2.5 g
   Monounsaturated Fat .....3.8 g
Cholesterol ....59 mg
Sodium ....321 mg
Total Carbohydrate ....21 g
   Dietary Fiber ....2 g
   Sugars ....4 g
Protein ....22 g

Salmon Croquettes with Yogurt-Horseradish Sauce

A zippy horseradish-infused yogurt sauce enlivens the down-home flavor of these croquettes. They're great hot, at room temperature, or chilled.

Serves 6; 1 salmon croquette and 2 tablespoons sauce per serving

YOGURT-HORSERADISH SAUCE

1/2 cup fat-free or low-fat plain yogurt
  2 tablespoons snipped fresh Italian (flat-leaf) parsley
  1 tablespoon prepared white horseradish
  1 tablespoon grated onion

SALMON CROQUETTES

    14.5-ounce can red or pink salmon, drained, bones discarded if desired and skin discarded
1/4 cup chopped red onion
1/2 cup chopped red bell pepper
1/3 cup crushed fat-free, no-salt-added crispbread
    Egg substitute equivalent to 1 egg, or 1 large egg
1/2 tablespoon snipped fresh dill weed or 1/2 teaspoon dried dill weed, crumbled
1/4 teaspoon pepper
  2 teaspoons canola oil

> **COOK'S TIP**
>
> *It's about as easy to crush an entire package of crispbread or crackers as it is to do just the amount a recipe calls for. Process several pieces in a food processor or blender until you have fine crumbs. Repeat the procedure with the remaining pieces. Use what you need, and freeze the rest in an airtight bag or a container with a tight-fitting lid.*

1   In a small bowl, stir together the sauce ingredients. Cover and refrigerate.

2   For the croquettes, put the salmon in a medium bowl. Flake the salmon. Stir in the remaining croquette ingredients except oil. Shape into 6 croquettes about 3 inches in diameter.

3   Heat a 12-inch skillet over medium-high heat. Pour in the oil and swirl to coat the bottom. When the oil is hot, cook the croquettes for 5 to 6 minutes, or until golden brown on both sides, turning once.

4   To serve, place the croquettes on plates. Spoon the sauce to the side or on top of the croquettes.

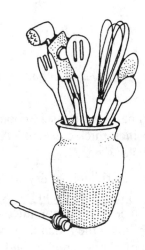

EXCHANGES

2 Lean Meat
1/2 Carbohydrate

Calories 133
   Calories from Fat 51
Total Fat..............................6 g
   Saturated Fat ....1.0 g
   Polyunsaturated Fat ....1.5 g
   Monounsaturated Fat .....2.7 g
Cholesterol ....25 mg
Sodium.........................351 mg
Total Carbohydrate...........6 g
   Dietary Fiber ....1 g
   Sugars ....2 g
Protein ....14 g

Salmon Baked with Cucumbers and Dill

Beautiful and light, this entrée is perfect for entertaining. The cucumbers will be slightly crisp after baking.

Serves 4; 3 ounces fish and 1/2 cup vegetables per serving

Vegetable oil spray
2 small cucumbers
1/2 small red onion, finely chopped
4 salmon fillets (about 4 ounces each)
2 tablespoons fresh lemon or lime juice
1/4 cup loosely packed snipped fresh dill weed
1/4 teaspoon salt
1/4 teaspoon pepper

1 Preheat the oven to 400°F. Lightly spray an 11 × 7 × 2-inch baking pan with vegetable oil spray.

2 Peel the cucumbers. Trim the ends. Cut each in half lengthwise. Scoop out and discard the seeds. Slice the cucumbers into 1/4-inch-thick crescents. Arrange the cucumbers and onion around the edges of the baking pan.

3 Rinse the fish and pat dry with paper towels. Place the fish in the center of the pan. Squeeze the lemon juice over the fish. Sprinkle the remaining ingredients over the fish, cucumbers, and onion.

4 Bake, uncovered, for 15 to 20 minutes, or until the fish flakes easily when tested with a fork and the vegetables are tender-crisp.

EXCHANGES

3 Lean Meat
1 Vegetable

Calories	206
Calories from Fat	88
Total Fat	10 g
Saturated Fat	1.7 g
Polyunsaturated Fat	2.2 g
Monounsaturated Fat	4.7 g
Cholesterol	77 mg
Sodium	207 mg
Total Carbohydrate	3 g
Dietary Fiber	1 g
Sugars	2 g
Protein	25 g

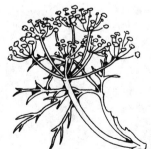

Roasted Cumin Snapper and Fresh Orange Salsa

Spicy citrus salsa makes a great accompaniment for baked fish, as here, and for grilled chicken and pork, too.

Serves 4; 3 ounces fish and 1/3 cup salsa per serving

FRESH ORANGE SALSA

  1 medium orange, cut into 1/2-inch pieces (about 1 cup) or 1 cup fresh pineapple chunks or pineapple chunks packed in their own juice
  1 small fresh jalapeño pepper, seeds and ribs discarded, minced
1/4 cup finely chopped radishes
1/4 cup snipped fresh cilantro
  1 teaspoon sugar
  1 teaspoon grated peeled gingerroot
  2 tablespoons fresh lemon juice

SNAPPER

   Vegetable oil spray
  4 red snapper or other mild fish fillets with skin (about 5 ounces each)
  2 teaspoons ground cumin
  1 teaspoon paprika
1/4 teaspoon salt

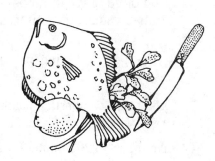

1 Preheat the oven to 350°F.

2 In a medium bowl, stir together the salsa ingredients. Set aside.

3 Lightly spray a nonstick baking sheet with vegetable oil spray. Rinse the fish and pat dry with paper towels. Place the fish on the baking sheet.

4 In a small bowl, stir together the cumin, paprika, and salt. Sprinkle over the fish. Spray lightly with vegetable oil spray.

5 Bake for 18 to 20 minutes, or until the fish flakes easily when tested with a fork.

6 To serve, place the fish on plates. Spoon the salsa on top or to the side of the fish.

EXCHANGES

4 Very Lean Meat
1/2 Fruit

Calories	169
Calories from Fat	20
Total Fat	2 g
Saturated Fat	0.4 g
Polyunsaturated Fat	0.7 g
Monounsaturated Fat	0.5 g
Cholesterol	48 mg
Sodium	210 mg
Total Carbohydrate	9 g
Dietary Fiber	2 g
Sugars	6 g
Protein	28 g

Creole-Sauced Snapper

Top tender baked fish fillets with a sauce of quickly cooked veggies, capers, and herbs and as much hot-pepper sauce as your taste buds can handle.

Serves 4; 3 ounces fish and 1/2 cup sauce per serving

Vegetable oil spray	1/4 cup finely chopped green
1 1/4 pounds red snapper fillets with skin	onions (green and white parts)
1 medium green bell pepper, chopped	2 tablespoons capers, rinsed and
1 large onion, chopped	drained
1 1/2 medium ribs of celery, chopped	1/4 cup snipped fresh parsley
1 teaspoon dried thyme, crumbled	2 tablespoons light tub margarine
1 medium garlic clove, minced	1/2 teaspoon red hot-pepper sauce,
1 cup diced grape tomatoes or cherry	or to taste
tomatoes (about 5 ounces)	3/4 teaspoon salt

1 Preheat the oven to 400°F.

2 Lightly spray a nonstick baking sheet with vegetable oil spray. Rinse the fish and pat dry with paper towels. Put the fish on the baking sheet.

3 Bake for 18 to 20 minutes, or until the fish flakes easily when tested with a fork.

4 Meanwhile, heat a 12-inch nonstick skillet over medium-high heat. Remove from the heat and lightly spray with vegetable oil spray (being careful not to spray near a gas flame). Cook the pepper, onion, celery, thyme, and garlic for 7 minutes, or until the onion is just tender.

5 Stir the tomatoes, green onions, and capers into the pepper mixture. Cook for 2 minutes, or until the tomatoes are soft, stirring constantly. Remove from the heat.

6 Stir the remaining ingredients into the pepper mixture. Cover to keep warm.

7 To serve, arrange the fish on a platter. Spoon the tomato mixture over the fish.

EXCHANGES

4 Very Lean Meat
1/2 Fruit

Calories	169
Calories from Fat	20
Total Fat	2 g
Saturated Fat	0.4 g
Polyunsaturated Fat	0.7 g
Monounsaturated Fat	0.5 g
Cholesterol	48 mg
Sodium	210 mg
Total Carbohydrate	9 g
Dietary Fiber	2 g
Sugars	6 g
Protein	28 g

Tuna-Macaroni Casserole with Tomatoes and Chickpeas

This meal-in-one is enhanced with fresh basil, cooked vegetables, and chickpeas.

Serves 4; 1 1/2 cups per serving

1 cup dried whole-wheat elbow macaroni or small shell pasta
Vegetable oil spray
2 teaspoons olive oil
1 medium onion, chopped
1 medium rib of celery, chopped
1 small red or green bell pepper, chopped
2 medium garlic cloves, minced
14.5-ounce can no-salt-added diced tomatoes, undrained
2 tablespoons no-salt-added tomato paste

1 tablespoon red wine vinegar
2 tablespoons snipped fresh basil or 2 teaspoons dried basil, crumbled
1/4 teaspoon salt
1/8 teaspoon cayenne
12-ounce can albacore tuna packed in spring or distilled water, rinsed and drained
1 cup no-salt-added chickpeas, rinsed and drained
3 tablespoons shredded Parmesan cheese

1 In a Dutch oven, cook the macaroni using the package directions, omitting the salt and oil. Drain in a colander, rinse with cold water, and drain again. Transfer to a large bowl.

2 Preheat the oven to 375°F. Lightly spray an 11 × 7 × 2-inch baking pan with vegetable oil spray.

3 Heat the Dutch oven over medium-high heat. Pour the olive oil into the Dutch oven and swirl to coat the bottom. Cook the onion, celery, bell pepper, and garlic for 3 to 4 minutes, or until the onion is tender, stirring occasionally.

4 Stir in the tomatoes, tomato paste, vinegar, basil, salt, and cayenne. Cook for 3 minutes, stirring frequently. Add to the pasta.

5 Stir the tuna and chickpeas into the pasta mixture. Spoon into the baking pan.

6 Bake, uncovered, for 10 minutes. Stir. Bake for 10 to 15 minutes, or until the casserole is very hot and most of the liquid is absorbed. Sprinkle with the Parmesan. Bake for 5 minutes, or until the cheese melts and is lightly golden.

EXCHANGES

2 Starch
2 Very Lean Meat
2 Vegetable
1/2 Fat

Calories	307
Calories from Fat	51
Total Fat	6 g
Saturated Fat	1.0 g
Polyunsaturated Fat	0.9 g
Monounsaturated Fat	2.5 g
Cholesterol	28 mg
Sodium	269 mg
Total Carbohydrate	43 g
Dietary Fiber	9 g
Sugars	10 g
Protein	24 g

Grilled Trout Amandine with Ginger and Orange

Ginger, thyme, and orange infuse mild trout fillets with flavor. Steamed red potatoes and asparagus or sugar snap peas make fine partners.

Serves 4; 3 ounces fish per serving

```
    Vegetable oil spray
  2 teaspoons canola oil
1/2 tablespoon minced peeled gingerroot
    or 1/2 teaspoon ground ginger
  1 teaspoon grated orange zest
  2 tablespoons fresh orange juice
1/2 tablespoon chopped fresh thyme
    or 1/2 teaspoon dried thyme, crumbled
1/4 teaspoon pepper
1/8 teaspoon salt
  4 rainbow trout fillets with skin
    (about 5 ounces each)
  3 tablespoons slivered almonds,
    dry-roasted
```

> **COOK'S TIP**
>
> *Trout are related to salmon and are a freshwater fish. Rainbow and steelhead are two popular varieties. They are sold both fresh and frozen year-round. When defrosting frozen trout or other seafood, follow the package directions carefully.*
>
> *Rinse the fish and dry thoroughly with several layers of paper towels. The fish will have retained a lot of water when frozen and should be thoroughly dry before you coat or cook it.*

1 Heat a ridged stovetop grill over medium-high heat. Remove from the heat and lightly spray with vegetable oil spray (being careful not to spray near a gas flame). If using an outdoor grill, lightly spray the grill rack with vegetable oil spray. Preheat the grill on medium high.

2 In a small bowl, stir together the oil, gingerroot, orange zest, orange juice, thyme, pepper, and salt.

3 Rinse the fish and pat dry with paper towels. Brush the oil mixture over the flesh side of the fish.

4 Grill the fish with the flesh side down for 3 minutes. Turn over and grill for 1 to 3 minutes, or until the fish flakes easily when tested with a fork.

5 To serve, remove the skin. Place the fish on plates. Sprinkle the almonds over each fillet.

EXCHANGES

4 Lean Meat
1/2 Fat

Calories	258
Calories from Fat	128
Total Fat	14 g
Saturated Fat	1.9 g
Polyunsaturated Fat	3.4 g
Monounsaturated Fat	7.7 g
Cholesterol	77 mg
Sodium	139 mg
Total Carbohydrate	2 g
Dietary Fiber	1 g
Sugars	1 g
Protein	29 g

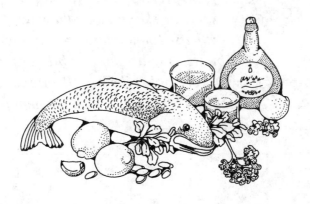

Tuna Kebabs

Whole-wheat couscous is a nice accompaniment for this meal on a stick.

Serves 6; 1 kebab per serving

MARINADE
       3 tablespoons pineapple juice
1 1/2 tablespoons light soy sauce
       1 tablespoon red wine vinegar or plain rice vinegar
       1 tablespoon water
       1 tablespoon honey
   1/4 cup chopped green onions (green and white parts)
       1 medium garlic clove, minced
   1/2 teaspoon ground ginger
   1/4 teaspoon pepper

KEBABS
       1 pound tuna without skin
         Vegetable oil spray
       1 small red or green bell pepper, cut into 12 squares
       1 small yellow summer squash or zucchini, cut into 12 slices
       1 small red onion, cut into 12 wedges
      12 1 1/2-inch cubes fresh pineapple
      12 grape tomatoes or cherry tomatoes

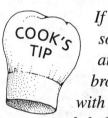

COOK'S TIP

If you prefer to broil the kebabs, soak the skewers in cold water for at least 10 minutes. Preheat the broiler. Lightly spray a broiler pan with vegetable oil spray. Broil the kebabs 4 to 5 inches from the heat for about 8 minutes.

1 In a large airtight plastic bag or glass baking dish, stir together the marinade ingredients. Remove and reserve 2 tablespoons marinade.

2 Rinse the fish and pat dry with paper towels. Cut the fish into 12 cubes. Add the fish to the marinade and turn to coat. Seal and refrigerate for 15 minutes to 1 hour. Remove the fish from the marinade; pat dry with paper towels. Discard this marinade.

3 Heat a large nonstick indoor grill pan over medium-high heat. Remove from the heat and lightly spray with vegetable oil spray (being careful not to spray near a gas flame). Return the pan to the heat for 1 minute.

4 Lightly spray six 12-inch bamboo or wooden skewers with vegetable oil spray. For each kebab, thread a skewer with 1 cube tuna, 1 wedge bell pepper, 1 slice squash, 1 wedge onion, 1 cube pineapple, and 1 tomato. Repeat. Baste with the 2 tablespoons reserved marinade.

5 Grill the kebabs for 7 to 9 minutes, or until the fish is cooked to the desired doneness and the squash and bell peppers are tender-crisp, turning once.

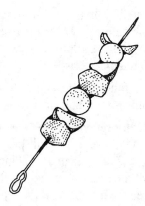

EXCHANGES

2 Lean Meat
1 Vegetable
1/2 Fruit

Calories 148
    Calories from Fat 35
Total Fat...........................4 g
    Saturated Fat ....0.9 g
    Polyunsaturated Fat ....1.2 g
    Monounsaturated Fat .....1.2 g
Cholesterol ....28 mg
Sodium.........................102 mg
Total Carbohydrate.........11 g
    Dietary Fiber ....2 g
    Sugars ....8 g
Protein ....18 g

Tuna and Vegetable Lasagna

This delicious lasagna combines vacuum-packed tuna with carrots, squash, sweet red peppers, a white sauce, and a topping of melted mozzarella and Parmesan.

Serves 6; 3 1/2 × 3 1/2-inch piece per serving

6 dried 10 × 2 1/2-inch lasagna noodles
Vegetable oil spray
1 medium zucchini or yellow summer squash, thinly sliced
1 medium red bell pepper, chopped
1 1/2 to 2 medium carrots, thinly sliced (about 1 cup)

10 3/4-ounce can reduced-fat, reduced-sodium condensed cream of mushroom soup
1/2 cup fat-free or light sour cream
1/4 teaspoon dried oregano, crumbled
7.6-ounce vacuum-sealed package light tuna
1 cup shredded part-skim mozzarella cheese
2 tablespoons shredded Parmesan cheese

1 Preheat the oven to 350°F.

2 Prepare the pasta using the package directions, omitting the salt and oil. Drain well.

3 Meanwhile, heat a large nonstick skillet over medium-high heat. Remove from the heat and lightly spray with vegetable oil spray (being careful not to spray near a gas flame). Put the zucchini, bell pepper, and carrots in the skillet. Lightly spray with vegetable oil spray. Cook for 6 minutes, or until the carrots are tender-crisp, stirring frequently.

4 In a medium bowl, stir together the soup, sour cream, and oregano.

5 Lightly spray an 11 × 7 × 2-inch baking dish with vegetable oil spray. To assemble, place 2 noodles in the baking dish. Spoon half the sauce over the noodles; spread evenly. Crumble half the tuna over the sauce. Spoon half the vegetable mixture over the tuna. Repeat with another layer of the noodles, tuna, and vegetable mixture, but do not add sauce to this layer. Arrange the remaining 2 noodles on top. Spread the remaining sauce over the noodles. Cover with aluminum foil.

6 Bake for 30 minutes, or until thoroughly heated. Sprinkle the mozzarella over the sauce. Bake, uncovered, for 10 minutes, or until the cheese melts. Remove from the oven. Sprinkle with the Parmesan. Let stand for 10 minutes before cutting.

EXCHANGES

1 Starch
2 Lean Meat
1 Vegetable
1/2 Carbohydrate

Calories 243
  Calories from Fat 49
Total Fat ....5 g
  Saturated Fat ....2.9 g
  Polyunsaturated Fat ....0.7 g
  Monounsaturated Fat .....1.4 g
Cholesterol ....29 mg
Sodium ....497 mg
Total Carbohydrate ....30 g
  Dietary Fiber ....3 g
  Sugars ....6 g
Protein ....19 g

Parsley Pesto Shrimp

Shrimp is tossed in a mixture of fresh lemon, parsley, and olive oil and served over rice to catch all the sauce.

Serves 4; 1/2 cup shrimp mixture and 1/2 cup cooked rice per serving

1/2 cup uncooked rice
  1 teaspoon grated lemon zest
  3 tablespoons fresh lemon juice
  2 tablespoons olive oil
1/4 cup minced fresh parsley
  1 medium garlic clove, minced
1/2 teaspoon salt
1/4 teaspoon crushed red pepper flakes
     Vegetable oil spray
  1 pound peeled raw medium shrimp
  1 medium lemon, quartered

1 Prepare the rice using the package directions, omitting the salt and margarine.

2 Meanwhile, in a small bowl, stir together the lemon zest, lemon juice, oil, parsley, garlic, salt, and red pepper flakes.

3 When the rice is almost ready, heat a large nonstick skillet over medium heat. Remove from the heat and lightly spray with vegetable oil spray (being careful not to spray near a gas flame). Cook the shrimp for 4 minutes, or until opaque in the center, stirring frequently. Remove from the heat. Gently stir in the lemon juice mixture.

4 To serve, spoon the rice onto plates. Spoon the shrimp mixture over the rice. Place 1 lemon quarter on each plate to squeeze over the shrimp.

EXCHANGES

1 1/2 Starch
2 Very Lean Meat
1 Fat

Calories	240
Calories from Fat	71
Total Fat	8 g
Saturated Fat	1.2 g
Polyunsaturated Fat	1.0 g
Monounsaturated Fat	5.2 g
Cholesterol	175 mg
Sodium	499 mg
Total Carbohydrate	21 g
Dietary Fiber	1 g
Sugars	1 g
Protein	21 g

Crab and Corn Cakes with Fresh Lemon

Fresh lemon brings out all the great flavors of these crab cakes.

Serves 4; 2 crab cakes per serving

Vegetable oil spray
1/2 medium red bell pepper, finely chopped
1/2 cup finely chopped green onions (green and white parts)
3/4 cup yellow cornmeal
1/4 cup all-purpose flour
1/2 teaspoon seafood seasoning blend
1/8 teaspoon cayenne
2 cups fresh crabmeat, picked over for shells and cartilage
1 cup frozen whole-kernel corn, thawed
1/4 cup snipped fresh parsley
1/3 cup fat-free or light mayonnaise dressing
Whites of 3 large eggs
1/4 cup fat-free milk
2 tablespoons fresh lemon juice
1/8 teaspoon salt
2 medium lemons, quartered

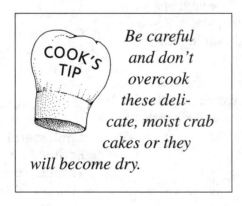

COOK'S TIP

Be careful and don't overcook these delicate, moist crab cakes or they will become dry.

1 Heat a 12-inch nonstick skillet over medium-high heat. Remove from the heat and lightly spray with vegetable oil spray (being careful not to spray near a gas flame). Cook the bell pepper and green onions for 3 minutes, or until tender, stirring frequently. Transfer to a large bowl to cool quickly.

2 Meanwhile, in a medium bowl, stir together the cornmeal, flour, seafood seasoning blend, and cayenne.

3 Stir the crabmeat, corn, parsley, mayonnaise, egg whites, milk, and lemon juice into the cooled vegetables. Stir in the cornmeal mixture until just blended.

4 Lightly spray the skillet with vegetable oil spray. Spoon 1/2 cup crab mixture into the skillet. Repeat three times. Flatten each patty to 1/2-inch thickness with a spatula. Cook for 3 minutes on each side. Set aside. Lightly spray the skillet with vegetable oil spray and repeat with the remaining crab mixture, making 4 more patties.

5 To serve, place 2 crab cakes on each plate. Sprinkle with salt. Place lemon wedges on each plate to squeeze over the crab cakes.

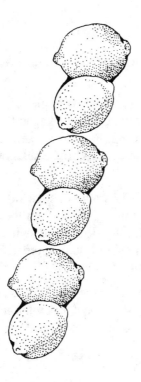

EXCHANGES

2 1/2 Starch
1 Very Lean Meat

Calories	249
Calories from Fat	12
Total Fat	1 g
Saturated Fat	0.2 g
Polyunsaturated Fat	0.5 g
Monounsaturated Fat	0.3 g
Cholesterol	34 mg
Sodium	517 mg
Total Carbohydrate	41 g
Dietary Fiber	4 g
Sugars	4 g
Protein	18 g

Skillet-Fried Oysters with Dijon Sour Cream

Follow these mess-free steps to a quick and easy entrée.

Serves 4; 8 oysters and 2 tablespoons sour cream mixture per serving

---

1/3 cup fat-free or light sour cream
1/2 tablespoon olive oil
  2 teaspoons Dijon mustard
1/4 teaspoon salt
1/4 teaspoon pepper
1/2 cup yellow cornmeal
  1 teaspoon paprika
  1 teaspoon Cajun seasoning blend (see Cook's Tip on Creole or Cajun seasoning, page 50)
32 medium oysters, drained (about 1 pint/1 pound)
  2 tablespoons canola oil

1 In a small bowl, whisk together the sour cream, olive oil, mustard, salt, and pepper. Set aside.

2 In a shallow dish or pie pan, stir together the cornmeal, paprika, and Cajun seasoning. Roll the oysters a few at a time to coat lightly. Shake off the excess.

3 Heat a 12-inch nonstick skillet over medium-high heat. Pour the vegetable oil into the skillet and swirl to coat the bottom. Cook the oysters for 4 minutes, turning frequently.

4 To serve, place 8 oysters on each plate. Serve with the sour cream mixture as a dipping sauce.

EXCHANGES

1 Lean Meat
1 Fat
1 1/2 Carbohydrate

Calories 207
  Calories from Fat 94
Total Fat..........................10 g
  Saturated Fat ....1.2 g
  Polyunsaturated Fat ....2.8 g
  Monounsaturated Fat .....5.6 g
Cholesterol ....31 mg
Sodium..........................408 mg
Total Carbohydrate........20 g
  Dietary Fiber ....1 g
  Sugars ....7 g
Protein ....7 g

Deep-South Shrimp Gumbo

The secret to excellent gumbo is browning the flour. It adds such depth to the flavor.

Serves 6; 1 cup gumbo and 1/2 cup rice per serving

1/4 cup all-purpose flour	1/4 teaspoon black pepper
2 teaspoons canola oil	14-ounce can low-fat, low-sodium chicken broth, divided use
1 medium green bell pepper, chopped	
1 large onion, chopped	
1 1/2 medium ribs of celery, chopped	1 pound peeled raw medium shrimp
14.5-ounce can stewed tomatoes (Cajun style preferred), undrained	1/2 teaspoon red hot-pepper sauce, or to taste
10-ounce package frozen cut okra	1/2 teaspoon salt
1 teaspoon dried thyme, crumbled	1 cup uncooked brown rice
2 bay leaves	

1 Heat a Dutch oven over medium-high heat. Cook the flour for 2 minutes, or until golden, stirring constantly with a flat spatula to prevent scorching. Pour the flour into a small bowl.

2 Pour the oil into the Dutch oven and swirl to coat the bottom. Cook the bell pepper, onion, and celery for 2 minutes, or until the onion is tender, stirring frequently.

3 Stir in the tomatoes, okra, thyme, bay leaves, black pepper, and all but 1/2 cup broth.

4 Stir the remaining broth into the flour to make a thick paste. Add the flour mixture to the tomato mixture, stirring until well blended. Bring to a boil. Reduce the heat and simmer, covered, for 30 minutes, or until the okra is very tender.

5 Stir in the shrimp. Simmer for 5 minutes, or until the shrimp is opaque in the center. Remove from the heat. Stir in the hot-pepper sauce and salt. Let stand, covered, for 30 minutes.

6 Meanwhile, prepare the rice using the package directions, omitting the salt and margarine.

7 To serve, reheat the gumbo over low heat if necessary. Spoon the rice into bowls. Ladle the gumbo over the rice.

EXCHANGES

2 Starch
1 Very Lean Meat
2 Vegetable
1/2 Fat

Calories 273
　Calories from Fat 35
Total Fat................................4 g
　Saturated Fat ....0.6 g
　Polyunsaturated Fat ....1.3 g
　Monounsaturated Fat .....1.5 g
Cholesterol ....117 mg
Sodium...........................527 mg
Total Carbohydrate.........40 g
　Dietary Fiber ....5 g
　Sugars ....7 g
Protein ....19 g

Poultry

Roast Chicken Breasts with Vegetable Medley

Chicken and vegetables roast in two pans and emerge from the oven at about the same time, making it easy to put a fantastic meal on the table.

Serves 4; 3 ounces chicken and 1 cup vegetables per serving

Vegetable oil spray

MARINADE
2 tablespoons fresh orange juice
2 teaspoons olive oil
2 medium garlic cloves, minced
1 tablespoon minced fresh thyme
   or 1 teaspoon dried thyme,
   crumbled
1/4 teaspoon pepper
1/8 teaspoon salt

VEGETABLES
1 medium leek (white part only)
1 medium sweet potato
1 medium white potato
1 medium red onion

1 cup baby carrots or 2 medium
   carrots
6 medium asparagus spears

CHICKEN
1 tablespoon fresh orange juice
1 medium garlic clove, minced
1/2 tablespoon minced fresh thyme
   or 1/2 teaspoon dried thyme,
   crumbled
1/4 teaspoon pepper
1/8 teaspoon salt
4 chicken breast halves with bone
   and skin (about 6 ounces each)

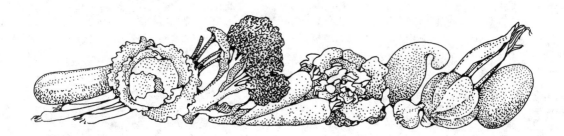

1 Preheat the oven to 400°F. Lightly spray a baking pan with vegetable oil spray. Place a rack in a roasting pan or another baking pan. Lightly spray the rack with vegetable oil spray.

2 In a large airtight plastic bag or glass baking dish, stir together the marinade ingredients. Set aside 2 teaspoons marinade.

3 Cut the leek in half lengthwise. Cut crosswise into 1/2-inch slices. Peel the sweet potato. Cut both potatoes like the leek. Cut the onion into 12 wedges. Slice the carrots if using medium size.

4 Put the prepared ingredients in the marinade. Turn to coat. Arrange the vegetables in a single layer in the baking pan. Bake for 15 minutes.

5 Meanwhile, trim the asparagus and cut in half crosswise. Brush with the reserved marinade. Set aside.

6 In a small bowl, stir together the remaining ingredients except the chicken. Loosen, but don't remove, the skin from the chicken. Using a basting or pastry brush or a spoon, spread one-fourth juice mixture under the skin of each breast. Put the chicken on the rack in the pan.

7 When the vegetables have cooked for 15 minutes, put the chicken in the oven. If the two pans do not fit on the same oven rack, use two racks, with the chicken on the upper rack. Roast for 25 minutes.

8 Add the asparagus to the pan with the vegetables, moving some of the other vegetables toward the sides of the pan so the asparagus will fit in a single layer. Roast the chicken and the vegetables for 10 to 12 minutes, or until the chicken is no longer pink in the center and all the vegetables are tender.

9 To serve, remove and discard the skin and all visible fat from the chicken. Place the chicken and vegetables on each plate.

EXCHANGES

1/2 Starch
3 Very Lean Meat
2 Vegetable
1 Fat

Calories 243
   Calories from Fat 51
Total Fat................................6 g
   Saturated Fat ....1.2 g
   Polyunsaturated Fat ....1.0 g
   Monounsaturated Fat .....2.9 g
Cholesterol ....75 mg
Sodium...........................231 mg
Total Carbohydrate.........18 g
   Dietary Fiber ....3 g
   Sugars ....10 g
Protein ....30 g

Chicken Stir-Fry with Snow Peas and Mixed Bell Peppers

Bell peppers provide a rainbow of colors in this attractive stir-fry. (See cover photo).

Serves 4; 3 ounces chicken and 3/4 cup vegetables per serving

1/2 cup low-fat, low-sodium chicken broth
2 tablespoons plain rice vinegar
2 tablespoons light soy sauce
1 teaspoon grated peeled gingerroot
2 medium garlic cloves, minced
1/4 teaspoon pepper
Vegetable oil spray
2 cups fresh or frozen snow peas or sugar snap peas, trimmed if fresh or thawed if frozen

1/3 cup chopped green onions (green and white parts)
1/2 medium red bell pepper, chopped
1/2 medium green bell pepper, chopped
1/2 medium yellow bell pepper, chopped
2 teaspoons canola oil
1 pound boneless, skinless chicken breasts, all visible fat discarded, cut into bite-size pieces
2 teaspoons cornstarch
1/4 cup water

1 In a small bowl, stir together the broth, vinegar, soy sauce, gingerroot, garlic, and pepper. Set aside.

2 Heat a large nonstick skillet or wok over medium-high heat. Remove from the heat and lightly spray with vegetable oil spray (being careful not to spray near a gas flame). Cook the snow peas, onions, and bell peppers for 4 to 5 minutes, or until tender-crisp, stirring occasionally. Transfer to a plate.

3 Pour the oil into the skillet and swirl to coat the bottom. Cook the chicken for 4 to 5 minutes, or until golden outside and no longer pink inside, stirring frequently.

4 Return the vegetables to the skillet. Stir in the broth mixture. Bring to a boil, still on medium high. Boil for 1 minute, stirring occasionally.

5 In a small bowl, whisk together the cornstarch and water until smooth. Pour into the skillet. Cook for 45 seconds to 1 minute, or until the mixture is thickened, stirring occasionally.

EXCHANGES

3 Very Lean Meat
2 Vegetable
1 Fat

Calories 203
  Calories from Fat 50
Total Fat...........................6 g
  Saturated Fat ....1.1 g
  Polyunsaturated Fat ....1.4 g
  Monounsaturated Fat .....2.6 g
Cholesterol ....69 mg
Sodium...........................363 mg
Total Carbohydrate.........10 g
  Dietary Fiber ....2 g
  Sugars ....4 g
Protein ....28 g

Tex-Mex Chicken Fingers

A favorite menu item at many restaurants, chicken fingers are easy to prepare at home. Serve with some crunchy raw veggies, such as carrot, celery, and bell pepper strips, and a low-fat dipping sauce on the side.

Serves 4; 3 ounces chicken per serving

1/3 cup fat-free or low-fat buttermilk	1/2 teaspoon ground cumin
1 teaspoon grated lime zest	1/2 teaspoon dried oregano, crumbled
1 tablespoon fresh lime juice	1/8 teaspoon cayenne
1/2 cup yellow cornmeal	Vegetable oil spray
2 tablespoons snipped fresh cilantro or Italian (flat-leaf) parsley	1 pound boneless, skinless chicken breasts or tenders, all visible fat discarded, cut into strips
1/2 teaspoon chili powder	

1 Preheat the oven to 400°F.

2 In a shallow dish or pie pan, whisk together the buttermilk, lime zest, and lime juice.

3 In another shallow dish or pie pan, stir together the cornmeal, cilantro, chili powder, cumin, oregano, and cayenne. Place the dishes side by side.

4 Lightly spray an 11 × 7 × 2-inch baking pan with vegetable oil spray. Set beside the cornmeal mixture.

5 Dip the chicken into the buttermilk mixture, turning to coat. Roll each piece in the cornmeal mixture, shaking off any excess. Arrange the chicken in a single layer on the baking pan. Lightly spray the top of the chicken with vegetable oil spray.

6 Bake, uncovered, for 20 to 25 minutes, or until the chicken is no longer pink in the center and the top coating is slightly crisp.

EXCHANGES

1 Starch
3 Very Lean Meat
1/2 Fat

Calories	208
Calories from Fat	31
Total Fat	3 g
Saturated Fat	0.9 g
Polyunsaturated Fat	0.8 g
Monounsaturated Fat	1.2 g
Cholesterol	69 mg
Sodium	86 mg
Total Carbohydrate	15 g
Dietary Fiber	2 g
Sugars	1 g
Protein	27 g

Oven-Fried Sesame-Ginger Chicken

This chicken is crunchy, moist, and juicy, all at the same time.

Serves 4; 3 ounces chicken per serving

White of 1 large egg
1 tablespoon cornstarch
2 tablespoons light soy or teriyaki sauce
1 tablespoon water
2 teaspoons canola oil
1 medium garlic clove, crushed

1 teaspoon grated peeled gingerroot
1/4 teaspoon pepper
1/3 cup sesame seeds
Vegetable oil spray
4 boneless, skinless chicken breast halves (about 4 ounces each), all visible fat discarded

1 Preheat the oven to 400°F.

2 In a shallow dish or pie pan, whisk together the egg white, cornstarch, soy sauce, water, oil, garlic, gingerroot, and pepper.

3 Pour the sesame seeds into another shallow dish or pie pan. Place the dishes side by side.

4 Lightly spray an 11 × 7 × 2-inch baking pan with vegetable oil spray. Set beside the sesame seeds.

5 Dip the chicken into the egg white mixture, turning to coat. Roll the chicken in the sesame seeds. Arrange the chicken in a single layer in the baking pan.

6 Bake for 25 to 30 minutes, or until the chicken is no longer pink in the center and the outside coating is crisp.

EXCHANGES

3 Very Lean Meat
2 Fat
1/2 Carbohydrate

Calories 242
  Calories from Fat 100
Total Fat...........................11 g
  Saturated Fat ....2.3 g
  Polyunsaturated Fat ....4.0 g
  Monounsaturated Fat .....4.6 g
Cholesterol ....69 mg
Sodium...........................360 mg
Total Carbohydrate...........6 g
  Dietary Fiber ....2 g
  Sugars ....2 g
Protein ....29 g

COOK'S TIP

The texture of cornstarch is a bit finer than that of flour, giving a more delicate finished product.

Baked Chicken Parmesan

You'll have to announce dinner only once when you're serving this favorite chicken dish. Whole-wheat or spinach pasta and a salad of assorted greens and cherry tomatoes would complete the meal very nicely.

Serves 4; 3 ounces chicken per serving

4 boneless, skinless chicken breast halves (about 4 ounces each) or 1 pound boneless, skinless turkey breast, all visible fat discarded
Egg substitute equivalent to 1 egg, or 1 large egg
1 tablespoon water
2 teaspoons olive oil

1/3 cup finely crushed reduced-sodium five-grain crispbread or whole-grain crackers
1/3 cup shredded Parmesan cheese
2 tablespoons minced fresh parsley
1/2 teaspoon ground oregano, crumbled
1/4 teaspoon pepper
Vegetable oil spray

1 Preheat the oven to 400°F.

2 Put the breasts with the smooth side up between two pieces of plastic wrap. If using turkey, cut crosswise into 4 pieces first. Using a tortilla press, the smooth side of a meat mallet, or a rolling pin, lightly flatten to a thickness of 1/4 inch, being careful not to tear the meat.

3 In a shallow dish or pie pan, whisk together the egg substitute, water, and oil.

4 In another shallow dish or pie pan, stir together the remaining ingredients except the vegetable oil spray. Place the dishes side by side.

5 Lightly spray a 13 × 9 × 2-inch baking pan with vegetable oil spray. Set beside the dishes.

6 Dip the chicken into the egg white mixture and turn to coat. Roll each piece in the crumb mixture, shaking off any excess. Arrange the chicken in a single layer on the baking sheet. Lightly spray the chicken with vegetable oil spray.

7 Bake, uncovered, for 15 to 18 minutes, or until the chicken is no longer pink in the center and the top coating is golden brown.

EXCHANGES

4 Very Lean Meat
1 Fat

Calories	200
Calories from Fat	66
Total Fat	7 g
Saturated Fat	2.1 g
Polyunsaturated Fat	1.1 g
Monounsaturated Fat	3.1 g
Cholesterol	74 mg
Sodium	144 mg
Total Carbohydrate	4 g
Dietary Fiber	1 g
Sugars	0 g
Protein	29 g

Cheese-Filled Oven-Fried Chicken

This is an all-purpose dish. Kids love it, but it is special enough for entertaining as well.

Serves 4; 1 chicken roll per serving

Vegetable oil spray
4 boneless, skinless chicken breast halves (about 4 ounces each), all visible fat discarded
2 slices of whole-wheat bread (about 1 ounce each), torn into small pieces
1 teaspoon dried basil
1/2 teaspoon dried oregano

1/4 teaspoon paprika
1/2 medium lemon
1/2 teaspoon dried basil, crumbled
1/4 teaspoon dried oregano, crumbled
1/4 cup snipped fresh parsley
4 3/4-ounce part-skim mozzarella cheese sticks (string cheese)
1/2 medium lemon
1/8 teaspoon salt

1 Preheat the oven to 400°F. Lightly spray a nonstick baking sheet with vegetable oil spray.

2 Place the breasts with the smooth side up between two pieces of plastic wrap. Using a tortilla press, the smooth side of a meat mallet, or a rolling pin, lightly flatten the breasts to a thickness of 1/4 inch, being careful not to tear the meat.

3 In a food processor or blender, process the bread, 1 teaspoon basil, 1/2 teaspoon oregano, and the paprika to the texture of coarse breadcrumbs. Set aside.

4 To assemble, put the chicken on the baking sheet. Squeeze the juice of half a lemon over the chicken. Sprinkle with the remaining 1/2 teaspoon basil and 1/4 teaspoon oregano. Place a cheese stick at one edge of each piece of chicken. Roll up jelly-roll fashion. Place with the seam side down on the baking sheet, leaving about 1/2 inch between the chicken rolls.

5 Squeeze the juice from the remaining lemon half over the rolls. Sprinkle with the breadcrumb mixture and salt. Lightly spray with vegetable oil spray.

6 Bake for 20 minutes, or until the chicken is no longer pink in the center.

EXCHANGES

1/2 Starch
4 Very Lean Meat
1 Fat

Calories 227
Calories from Fat 62
Total Fat.............................7 g
Saturated Fat ....3.2 g
Polyunsaturated Fat ....0.9 g
Monounsaturated Fat .....2.2 g
Cholesterol ....81 mg
Sodium..........................313 mg
Total Carbohydrate..........8 g
Dietary Fiber ....1 g
Sugars ....1 g
Protein ....32 g

Chicken and Asparagus Toss

You'll appreciate how easy this dish is to prepare—it can be on the table in minutes—and how good it tastes.

Serves 4; scant 1 cup chicken mixture and 1/2 cup rice per serving

1/2 cup uncooked rice
2 tablespoons olive oil
1/2 tablespoon grated lemon zest
2 to 3 tablespoons fresh lemon juice
1/2 teaspoon salt
1/2 cup water
6 ounces asparagus, trimmed, cut into 2-inch pieces

Vegetable oil spray
1 pound boneless, skinless chicken breasts, all visible fat discarded, cut into bite-size pieces
1/2 tablespoon dried dill weed, crumbled
1 medium garlic clove, minced

1 Prepare the rice using the package directions, omitting the salt and margarine.

2 Meanwhile, in a small bowl, stir together the oil, lemon zest, lemon juice, and salt. Set aside.

3 In a 12-inch nonstick skillet, bring the water to a boil over high heat. Add the asparagus and return to a boil. Reduce the heat and simmer, covered, for 2 minutes, or until just tender-crisp. Drain and set aside.

4 Dry the skillet with paper towels. Lightly spray the skillet with vegetable oil spray (being careful not to spray near a gas flame). Cook the chicken and dill weed for 4 minutes, or until the chicken is no longer pink in the center, stirring frequently.

5 Stir the asparagus and garlic into the chicken. Cook for 30 seconds, or until the asparagus is heated, stirring constantly. Remove from the heat. Stir in the lemon mixture to coat.

6 To serve, spoon the rice onto a platter. Spoon the chicken mixture over the rice.

EXCHANGES

1 Starch	3 Very Lean Meat
1 1/2 Fat	1 Vegetable

Calories 287
 Calories from Fat 89
Total Fat..........................10 g
 Saturated Fat ....1.7 g
 Polyunsaturated Fat ....1.2 g
 Monounsaturated Fat .....6.0 g
Cholesterol ....69 mg
Sodium...........................357 mg
Total Carbohydrate.........21 g
 Dietary Fiber ....1 g
 Sugars ....1 g
Protein ....27 g

Chicken with Country Gravy

Preparing a home-cooked meal, especially if the main dish is as easy as this one, is a very soothing way to dissolve the stress of the day.

Serves 4; 3 ounces chicken and 2 tablespoons gravy per serving

3 tablespoons all-purpose flour	Vegetable oil spray
1 cup low-fat, low-sodium chicken broth	4 boneless, skinless chicken breast halves (about 4 ounces each), all visible fat discarded
1/4 teaspoon paprika	
1/4 teaspoon garlic powder	2 tablespoons light tub margarine
1/4 teaspoon poultry seasoning	1/4 teaspoon salt

1 Heat a 12-inch nonstick skillet over medium-high heat. Cook the flour for 1 to 2 minutes, or until beginning to lightly brown, stirring constantly (a flat spatula works well). Remove from the heat and spread on a plate to cool.

2 Put the broth, paprika, garlic powder, poultry seasoning, and cooled flour in a jar with a tight-fitting lid. Cover and shake until completely blended.

3 Lightly spray the skillet with vegetable oil spray (being careful not to spray near a gas flame). Cook the chicken with the smooth side down for 2 minutes, or until beginning to brown. Put on a plate.

4 Reduce the heat to medium. Put the margarine in the skillet and let it melt. Pour in the broth mixture. Scrape the bottom and sides of the skillet to loosen any particles.

5 Add the chicken and salt. Spoon the sauce over the chicken. Reduce the heat and simmer, covered, for 10 minutes, or until the chicken is no longer pink in the center, stirring frequently.

6 To serve, place the chicken on a platter. Pour the sauce over the chicken.

EXCHANGES

1/2 Starch
3 Very Lean Meat
1 Fat

Calories 184
  Calories from Fat 51
Total Fat...............................6 g
  Saturated Fat ....0.9 g
  Polyunsaturated Fat ....1.3 g
  Monounsaturated Fat .....2.4 g
Cholesterol ....70 mg
Sodium..........................279 mg
Total Carbohydrate...........5 g
  Dietary Fiber ....0 g
  Sugars ....0 g
Protein ....27 g

Seared Chicken with Strawberry Salsa

Strawberries, mango, peaches—take your pick! Strawberries are the most unusual for salsa, but all three choices are winners.

Serves 4; 3 ounces chicken and 1/2 cup salsa per serving

CHICKEN
1/2 teaspoon paprika
1/4 teaspoon ground allspice or cumin
1/4 teaspoon salt
1/4 teaspoon black pepper
4 boneless, skinless chicken breast halves (about 4 ounces each), all visible fat discarded

SALSA
1 cup diced strawberries, mango, or peeled peaches

1 medium poblano pepper, seeded and ribs discarded, diced, or 3/4 medium green bell pepper, chopped
1/2 cup finely chopped red onion
1/4 cup chopped fresh mint or snipped fresh cilantro
2 tablespoons fresh lemon juice
1 tablespoon sugar
1/8 teaspoon crushed red pepper flakes

Vegetable oil spray
2 teaspoons canola oil

1 In a small bowl, stir together the paprika, allspice, salt, and black pepper. Sprinkle over the smooth side of the chicken pieces, pressing with your fingertips so the mixture adheres. Let stand for 10 minutes.

2 Meanwhile, in a medium bowl, stir together the salsa ingredients.

3 Heat a 12-inch nonstick skillet over medium-high heat. Remove from the heat and lightly spray with vegetable oil spray (being careful not to spray near a gas flame). Pour in the oil and swirl to coat the bottom. Cook the chicken with the smooth side down for 4 minutes. Turn over and cook for 4 to 5 minutes, or until no longer pink in the center.

4 To serve, put the chicken on plates and spoon the salsa on the side.

EXCHANGES

3 Very Lean Meat
1 Vegetable
1/2 Fruit
1 Fat

Calories	195
Calories from Fat	49
Total Fat	5 g
Saturated Fat	1.0 g
Polyunsaturated Fat	1.4 g
Monounsaturated Fat	2.4 g
Cholesterol	69 mg
Sodium	210 mg
Total Carbohydrate	10 g
Dietary Fiber	2 g
Sugars	7 g
Protein	26 g

Chicken and Noodles with Alfredo-Style Sauce

You really need to use fresh garlic for this dish. It is the key to the excellence of the sauce.

Serves 4; 1 1/3 cups per serving

6 ounces dried no-yolk egg noodles
1/4 cup light tub cream cheese
1/4 cup fat-free or light sour cream
1/4 cup fat-free milk
1 medium garlic clove
1/2 teaspoon salt
1/4 teaspoon pepper
Vegetable oil spray

1 pound boneless, skinless chicken breasts or tenderloins, all visible fat discarded, cut into thin strips
1/4 cup minced green onions (green and white parts)
2 tablespoons shredded Parmesan cheese
Pepper to taste (optional)

1 Prepare the noodles using the package directions, omitting the salt and oil. Drain well.

2 Meanwhile, in a food processor or blender, process the cream cheese, sour cream, milk, garlic, salt, and 1/4 teaspoon pepper until smooth.

3 Heat a 12-inch nonstick skillet over medium heat. Remove from the heat and lightly spray with vegetable oil spray (being careful not to spray near a gas flame). Cook the chicken for 5 minutes, or until no longer pink in the center, stirring frequently.

4 Stir in the cream cheese mixture. Cook for 30 seconds. Stir in the noodles. Remove from the heat.

5 To serve, sprinkle with the green onions, Parmesan, and pepper.

EXCHANGES

2 1/2 Starch
4 Very Lean Meat
1/2 Fat

Calories	354
Calories from Fat	58
Total Fat	6 g
Saturated Fat	2.8 g
Polyunsaturated Fat	0.9 g
Monounsaturated Fat	2.2 g
Cholesterol	80 mg
Sodium	497 mg
Total Carbohydrate	36 g
Dietary Fiber	2 g
Sugars	5 g
Protein	35 g

Skillet Chicken with Lime Barbecue Sauce

Of all the ways you've jazzed up barbecue sauce, you've probably never added limeade. Go ahead and wake up your taste buds with this quick and easy dish!

Serves 4; 3 ounces chicken and about 1 1/2 tablespoons sauce per serving

4 boneless, skinless chicken breast halves (about 4 ounces each), all visible fat discarded
Vegetable oil spray
1/4 cup barbecue sauce
1/4 cup frozen limeade concentrate
1/4 teaspoon crushed red pepper flakes
1/2 teaspoon grated peeled gingerroot (optional)

1 Heat a 12-inch nonstick skillet over medium-high heat. Remove from the heat and lightly spray with vegetable oil spray (being careful not to spray near a gas flame). Cook the chicken for 4 minutes on each side, or until no longer pink in the center. Place on plates.

2 In a small bowl, stir together the remaining ingredients except the gingerroot. Stir into the pan juices. Cook for 1 minute, or until reduced slightly, stirring constantly. Remove from the heat.

3 Stir the gingerroot into the sauce. Spoon over the chicken.

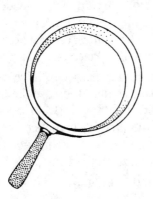

EXCHANGES

3 Very Lean Meat
1 Carbohydrate

Calories	178
Calories from Fat	28
Total Fat	3 g
Saturated Fat	0.9 g
Polyunsaturated Fat	0.7 g
Monounsaturated Fat	1.1 g
Cholesterol	69 mg
Sodium	187 mg
Total Carbohydrate	11 g
Dietary Fiber	0 g
Sugars	10 g
Protein	25 g

Citrus Chicken

If one citrus juice is good, three must be terrific! One taste of this chicken and you'll know what we mean.

Serves 4; 3 ounces chicken and 2 tablespoons sauce per serving

---

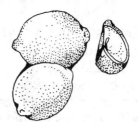

  1 cup grapefruit juice
1/4 cup frozen orange juice concentrate
  2 tablespoons honey
  1 tablespoon fresh lemon juice
  2 teaspoons grated peeled gingerroot
1/8 teaspoon crushed red pepper flakes
  4 boneless, skinless chicken breast halves (about 4 ounces each)
     Vegetable oil spray
  1 tablespoon light tub margarine
1/4 teaspoon salt

1 In a medium nonmetallic bowl, stir together the grapefruit juice, orange juice concentrate, honey, lemon juice, gingerroot, and red pepper flakes. Remove and set aside 1 cup juice mixture.

2 Add the chicken pieces to the juice mixture remaining in the bowl. Turn the chicken to coat. Let marinate for 15 minutes, turning occasionally.

3 Heat a 12-inch nonstick skillet over medium heat. Remove from the heat and lightly spray with vegetable oil spray (being careful not to spray near a gas flame). Remove the chicken from the marinade; discard the marinade. Cook the chicken for 5 minutes. Turn over and cook for 5 to 6 minutes, or until no longer pink in the center. Place on a plate.

4 Stir the reserved 1 cup juice mixture into the pan residue. Increase the heat to high and bring to a boil. Boil for 3 minutes, or until the mixture is reduced to 1/2 cup, scraping the bottom and sides of the pan. Remove from the heat.

5 Stir in the margarine and salt. Pour over the chicken.

EXCHANGES

3 Very Lean Meat
1 Fruit
1/2 Fat

Calories	192
Calories from Fat	37
Total Fat	4 g
Saturated Fat	0.8 g
Polyunsaturated Fat	0.9 g
Monounsaturated Fat	1.6 g
Cholesterol	69 mg
Sodium	229 mg
Total Carbohydrate	12 g
Dietary Fiber	0 g
Sugars	10 g
Protein	26 g

Creole Drums

Serve this in shallow soup bowls so you don't miss out on any of the great-tasting sauce.

Serves 4; 2 drumsticks and 1 cup vegetable mixture per serving

Vegetable oil spray
8 skinless chicken drumsticks with bone, all visible fat discarded (about 2 pounds)
1 large onion, chopped
1 medium green bell pepper, chopped
14.5-ounce can diced tomatoes with green peppers and onions, undrained
10 ounces fresh or frozen cut okra, cut into 1/2-inch slices if fresh
1 teaspoon low-sodium Worcestershire sauce
1/2 teaspoon dried thyme, crumbled
1/4 teaspoon red hot-pepper sauce
1/8 teaspoon salt

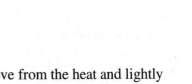

1 Heat a Dutch oven over medium-high heat. Remove from the heat and lightly spray with vegetable oil spray (being careful not to spray near a gas flame). Cook the chicken for about 4 minutes, or until browned on all sides, turning frequently. Place the chicken on a plate.

2 Stir the onion and bell pepper into the pan juices. Cook for 3 minutes, or until beginning to lightly brown on the edges, stirring frequently.

3 Gently stir in the chicken with any accumulated juices and the remaining ingredients except the salt. Bring to a boil, still over medium-high heat. Reduce the heat and simmer, covered, for 40 minutes, or until the chicken is no longer pink in the center and the okra is very tender. Remove from the heat.

4 To serve, put the chicken in soup bowls. Stir the salt into the tomato mixture. Pour over the chicken.

EXCHANGES

3 Lean Meat
3 Vegetable

Calories 239
  Calories from Fat 47
Total Fat............................5 g
  Saturated Fat ....1.3 g
  Polyunsaturated Fat ....1.3 g
  Monounsaturated Fat .....1.6 g
Cholesterol ....78 mg
Sodium..........................547 mg
Total Carbohydrate.........20 g
  Dietary Fiber ....5 g
  Sugars ....12 g
Protein ....27 g

Chicken Pot Pie

The whole-wheat crust for this bountiful dish is so simple to make—no rolling required! It is more like a thick batter that is spread over the pie. Stick with the traditional combo of carrots, green beans, and corn, or branch out and try something unexpected.

Serves 6; 1 1/2 cups per serving

Vegetable oil spray
1-pound package unseasoned frozen mixed vegetables, any combination
2/3 cup low-fat, low-sodium chicken broth
2 teaspoons cornstarch
2 tablespoons water
1 pound cooked boneless, skinless chicken breasts, chopped

2/3 cup fat-free or low-fat buttermilk
Egg substitute equivalent to 1 egg, or 1 large egg
1 tablespoon light stick margarine, melted and cooled
2/3 cup whole-wheat pastry flour
1/3 cup cornmeal
1/2 tablespoon baking powder
1/4 teaspoon salt
2 tablespoons minced fresh parsley

1 Preheat the oven to 425°F. Lightly spray an 11 × 7 × 2-inch glass baking pan with vegetable oil spray.

2 In a medium saucepan, cook the frozen vegetables using the package directions, omitting the salt and margarine. Drain. Set the vegetables aside.

3 In the same saucepan, bring the broth to a boil over medium-high heat.

4 Put the cornstarch in a small bowl. Add the water, stirring to dissolve. Stir into the hot broth. Cook for 1 minute, or until the mixture comes to a boil and thickens, stirring frequently. Remove the saucepan from the heat.

5 Stir in the chicken and vegetables. Pour into the baking pan.

6 For the crust, in a medium bowl, whisk together the buttermilk, egg substitute, and margarine. Stir in the remaining ingredients until just combined. Spread the batter over the chicken mixture.

7 Bake, uncovered, for 30 to 35 minutes, or until the crust is golden brown and a toothpick inserted in the center of the crust comes out clean.

EXCHANGES

1 1/2 Starch	3 Very Lean Meat
1/2 Fat	1 Vegetable

Calories	261
Calories from Fat	41
Total Fat	5 g
Saturated Fat	1.1 g
Polyunsaturated Fat	1.2 g
Monounsaturated Fat	1.5 g
Cholesterol	66 mg
Sodium	338 mg
Total Carbohydrate	24 g
Dietary Fiber	4 g
Sugars	3 g
Protein	29 g

Roast Turkey with Orange-Spice Rub

An aromatic spice rub cooks into a rich paste that penetrates deep into the turkey breast. Don't serve this dish just for the winter holidays. It is great year-round. If you're lucky, you'll have turkey left over to use in Cranberry-Pecan Turkey Salad (page 49).

Serves 11; 3 ounces turkey per serving

Vegetable oil spray
1 tablespoon grated orange zest
1/2 teaspoon ground cinnamon
1/2 teaspoon ground cumin
1/2 teaspoon paprika
1/4 teaspoon ground allspice, 1/4 teaspoon ground nutmeg, or 1/8 teaspoon ground cloves
1/4 teaspoon black pepper
1/4 teaspoon salt
1/8 teaspoon cayenne
5-pound whole turkey breast with skin and bone in

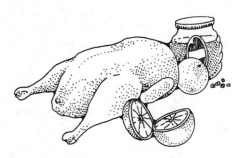

1 Preheat the oven to 325°F. Lightly spray a roasting pan and a baking rack with vegetable oil spray.

2 In a small bowl, stir together the remaining ingredients except the turkey.

3 Using your fingertips, loosen but don't remove the skin from the turkey breast. Rub the orange zest mixture evenly over the breast. Cover it with the skin. Put the turkey on the rack in the roasting pan.

4 Roast the turkey, uncovered, for 1 hour 45 minutes, or until a meat thermometer inserted in the thickest part registers 170°F. Be sure the thermometer doesn't touch the bone.

5 Let the turkey stand for 15 minutes. Discard the skin and all visible fat before slicing the turkey.

EXCHANGES

3 Very Lean Meat

Calories 116
  Calories from Fat 6
Total Fat...........................1 g
  Saturated Fat ....0.3 g
  Polyunsaturated Fat ....0.3 g
  Monounsaturated Fat ....0 g
Cholesterol ....69 mg
Sodium...........................98 mg
Total Carbohydrate..........0 g
  Dietary Fiber ....0 g
  Sugars ....0 g
Protein ....26 g

Turkey Marsala

Both family and friends will rave about the marvelous flavor marsala, thyme, and lemon impart to this dish. Try it with a whole-grain pasta and steamed broccoli.

Serves 4; 3 ounces turkey per serving

3 tablespoons cornstarch
1 teaspoon dried thyme, crumbled
1 teaspoon grated lemon zest
1/4 teaspoon pepper
1 pound boneless, skinless turkey breast, cut crosswise into 4 slices, or turkey breast cutlets, all visible fat discarded

2 teaspoons canola oil
1/3 cup dry marsala or dry red wine (regular or nonalcoholic)
1/3 cup low-fat, low-sodium chicken broth
2 tablespoons fresh lemon juice
2 tablespoons chopped fresh Italian (flat-leaf) parsley

1 In a pie pan or shallow dish, stir together the cornstarch, thyme, lemon zest, and pepper. Lightly dust both sides of the turkey, shaking off the excess.

2 Heat a medium nonstick skillet over medium-high heat. Pour in the oil and swirl to coat the bottom. Cook the turkey for 6 to 8 minutes, or until lightly browned and no longer pink in the center, turning once. Transfer the turkey to a platter. Cover with aluminum foil to keep warm.

3 Stir the remaining ingredients into the skillet. Increase the heat to high and bring to a boil. Cook for 1 minute, or until the sauce is reduced slightly, using a wooden spoon to scrape up any browned bits on the bottom of the pan.

4 To serve, spoon the sauce over the turkey.

EXCHANGES

3 Very Lean Meat
1/2 Fat
1/2 Carbohydrate

Calories	173
Calories from Fat	27
Total Fat	3 g
Saturated Fat	0.5 g
Polyunsaturated Fat	1.0 g
Monounsaturated Fat	1.4 g
Cholesterol	73 mg
Sodium	60 mg
Total Carbohydrate	5 g
Dietary Fiber	0 g
Sugars	0 g
Protein	27 g

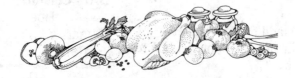

Turkey Loaf

Serve this moist, vegetable-flecked turkey loaf with steamed green beans or broccoli for a colorful and delicious meal. If there are any leftovers, you can make great cold turkey-loaf sandwiches on whole-grain bread or rolls.

Serves 4; 2 slices per serving

Vegetable oil spray
1/2 cup no-salt-added tomato sauce
Egg substitute equivalent to 1 egg, or 1 large egg
2 teaspoons balsamic or red wine vinegar
1/2 cup diced onion
1 medium rib of celery, diced
1/2 medium red or green bell pepper, diced

1/3 cup finely crushed fat-free, no-salt-added whole-grain crackers
1/2 teaspoon dried thyme, crumbled
1/4 teaspoon salt
1/4 teaspoon pepper
1 pound lean ground turkey breast, skin removed before grinding
1/3 cup no-salt-added tomato sauce
1/2 tablespoon honey

1 Preheat the oven to 350°F. Lightly spray a broiler pan and rack or a roasting pan and baking rack with vegetable oil spray.

2 In a large bowl, stir together 1/2 cup tomato sauce, egg substitute, vinegar, onion, celery, bell pepper, cracker crumbs, thyme, salt, and pepper.

3 Stir in the turkey. You'll get the best results by mixing with your hands, but you can use a spoon if you prefer. Shape the mixture into a loaf about 8 1/4 × 4 1/2 × 2 1/4 inches and slide it onto the rack in the pan.

4 Bake for 55 minutes.

5 Meanwhile, in a small bowl, stir together 1/3 cup tomato sauce and honey. Spread over the top of the turkey loaf.

6 Bake for 15 to 20 minutes, or until the turkey loaf is cooked through and the topping is hot.

EXCHANGES

3 Very Lean Meat
1 Carbohydrate

Calories	178
Calories from Fat	10
Total Fat	1 g
Saturated Fat	0 g
Polyunsaturated Fat	0 g
Monounsaturated Fat	0 g
Cholesterol	64 mg
Sodium	261 mg
Total Carbohydrate	14 g
Dietary Fiber	2 g
Sugars	8 g
Protein	28 g

Stir-Fry Turkey Strips with Broccoli, Green Onions, and Water Chestnuts

You'll get rid of the phone number of your favorite Chinese take-out restaurant after you taste this stir-fry. Serve it with fluffy brown rice and fresh fruit salad.

Serves 4; 3 ounces turkey and 3/4 cup vegetables per serving

- 1/2 cup pineapple juice
- 2 tablespoons hoisin sauce
- 1 teaspoon toasted sesame oil
- 1/2 teaspoon ground cardamom
- 1/4 teaspoon crushed red pepper flakes
  Vegetable oil spray
  1 pound boneless, skinless turkey tenderloins, all visible fat discarded, cut into thin strips
- 1/2 tablespoon canola oil
- 2 cups small broccoli florets
- 1 medium rib of celery, sliced
- 1/2 cup sliced green onions (green and white parts)
- 1 1/2 cups sliced exotic mushrooms—such as straw, enoki, or wood ear— or button mushrooms
- 2 medium garlic cloves, minced
  8-ounce can sliced water chestnuts, rinsed and drained
- 2 teaspoons cornstarch
- 1/4 cup pineapple juice

COOK'S TIP

Water chestnuts grow underground and resemble muddy flower bulbs. Although most home cooks use the canned variety, you may want to experiment with fresh water chestnuts, available in Asian food markets. A good source of fiber, water chestnuts add crunch to stir-fries, salads, and side dishes.

1. In a small bowl, stir together 1/2 cup pineapple juice, hoisin sauce, sesame oil, cardamom, and red pepper flakes.

2. Heat a large nonstick skillet or wok over medium-high heat. Remove from the heat and lightly spray with vegetable oil spray (being careful not to spray near a gas flame). Cook the turkey for 5 to 7 minutes, or until no longer pink in the center, stirring frequently. Transfer the turkey to a plate. Lightly cover with aluminum foil to keep warm.

3. Reduce the heat to medium. Pour the vegetable oil into the same skillet and swirl to coat the bottom. Cook the broccoli, celery, and green onions for 3 to 4 minutes, or until the broccoli is tender-crisp, stirring frequently.

4. Stir in the mushrooms and garlic. Cook for 2 to 4 minutes, or until the mushrooms begin to soften.

5. Stir in the turkey, water chestnuts, and pineapple juice mixture. Increase the heat to medium high and bring to a boil.

6. Put the cornstarch in a small bowl. Add the remaining 1/4 cup pineapple juice, stirring to dissolve. Stir into the turkey mixture. Cook for 1 minute, or until the mixture comes to a boil and thickens, stirring frequently.

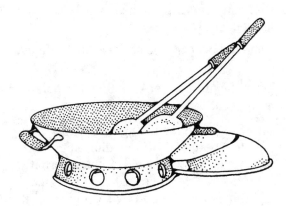

EXCHANGES

3 Very Lean Meat
2 Vegetable
1/2 Fruit
1/2 Fat

Calories 225
    Calories from Fat 34
Total Fat..............................4 g
    Saturated Fat ....0.6 g
    Polyunsaturated Fat ....1.4 g
    Monounsaturated Fat .....1.5 g
Cholesterol ....73 mg
Sodium.........................230 mg
Total Carbohydrate.........18 g
    Dietary Fiber ....3 g
    Sugars ....11 g
Protein ....30 g

Turkey Chili

Fresh jalapeño pepper and crushed red pepper flakes will get your attention when you sample this chili.

Serves 4; 1 1/2 cups per serving

1/2 tablespoon canola oil	1 pound lean ground turkey breast, skin discarded before grinding
1/2 cup chopped red onion	
2 medium garlic cloves, minced	14.5-ounce can no-salt-added diced tomatoes, undrained
1 teaspoon ground cumin	
1 teaspoon dried oregano, crumbled	8-ounce can no-salt-added tomato sauce
1 teaspoon chopped fresh jalapeño pepper, seeds and ribs discarded	1 cup low-fat, low-sodium chicken broth
1/4 teaspoon crushed red pepper flakes	15-ounce can no-salt-added kidney beans, rinsed and drained

1 In a medium nonstick saucepan, heat the oil over medium heat. Cook the onion and garlic for about 2 minutes, or until tender-crisp.

2 Stir in the cumin, oregano, jalapeño, and red pepper flakes. Cook for 1 minute, stirring constantly.

3 Increase the heat to medium high. Stir in the turkey. Cook for 3 to 4 minutes, or until browned on the outside, stirring frequently.

4 Stir in the remaining ingredients. Bring to a boil, still over medium-high heat. Reduce the heat and simmer, partially covered, for 30 minutes, or until the liquid has reduced by about one-third.

EXCHANGES

1 Starch	4 Very Lean Meat
2 Vegetable	

Calories	271
Calories from Fat	31
Total Fat	3 g
Saturated Fat	0.5 g
Polyunsaturated Fat	1.1 g
Monounsaturated Fat	1.4 g
Cholesterol	65 mg
Sodium	139 mg
Total Carbohydrate	27 g
Dietary Fiber	8 g
Sugars	10 g
Protein	33 g

COOK'S TIP

Hot chili peppers contain oils that can burn your skin, lips, and eyes. Wear rubber gloves or wash your hands thoroughly with warm, soapy water immediately after handling peppers.

Meats

Company Roast Tenderloin

This simply prepared roast is perfect for formal entertaining. The high heat of the oven sears the mustard crust on the roast, locking in the flavorful juices.

Serves 8; 3 ounces meat per serving

3 tablespoons country Dijon or coarse-grained mustard
2 tablespoons chopped fresh thyme or 2 teaspoons dried thyme, crumbled
4 medium garlic cloves, minced
1/2 teaspoon salt
1/2 teaspoon pepper
  Vegetable oil spray
  2-pound beef tenderloin, all visible fat and silver skin discarded

1 Preheat the oven to 450°F.

2 In a small bowl, stir together the mustard, thyme, garlic, salt, and pepper.

3 Spray a shallow roasting pan with vegetable oil spray. Put the roast in the pan. Spread the mustard mixture over the roast.

4 Bake, uncovered, for 25 to 30 minutes, or until desired doneness. Transfer the roast to a cutting board. Lightly cover with aluminum foil. Let stand for 10 to 15 minutes.

5 To serve, cut the roast crosswise into thin slices.

EXCHANGES

3 Lean Meat

Calories	159
Calories from Fat	65
Total Fat	7 g
Saturated Fat	2.8 g
Polyunsaturated Fat	0.3 g
Monounsaturated Fat	2.9 g
Cholesterol	60 mg
Sodium	326 mg
Total Carbohydrate	2 g
Dietary Fiber	0 g
Sugars	1 g
Protein	20 g

COOK'S TIP

The tough membrane sometimes found on the outside of tenderloin and flank steak is called silver skin. It should be removed before the meat is cooked. Slide a sharp knife under the silver skin, and cut it off. Leaving the silver skin on causes the meat to curl up during cooking.

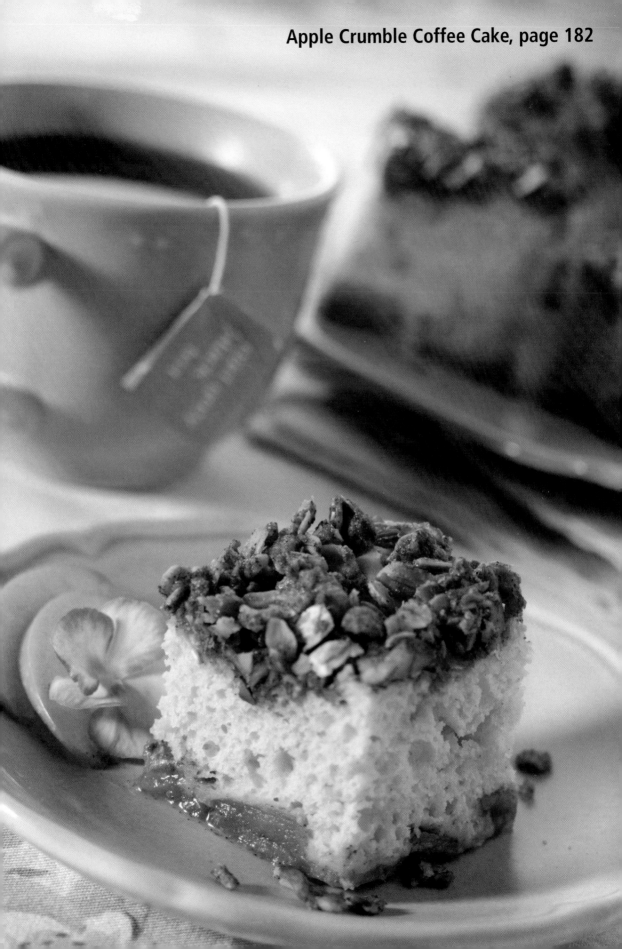

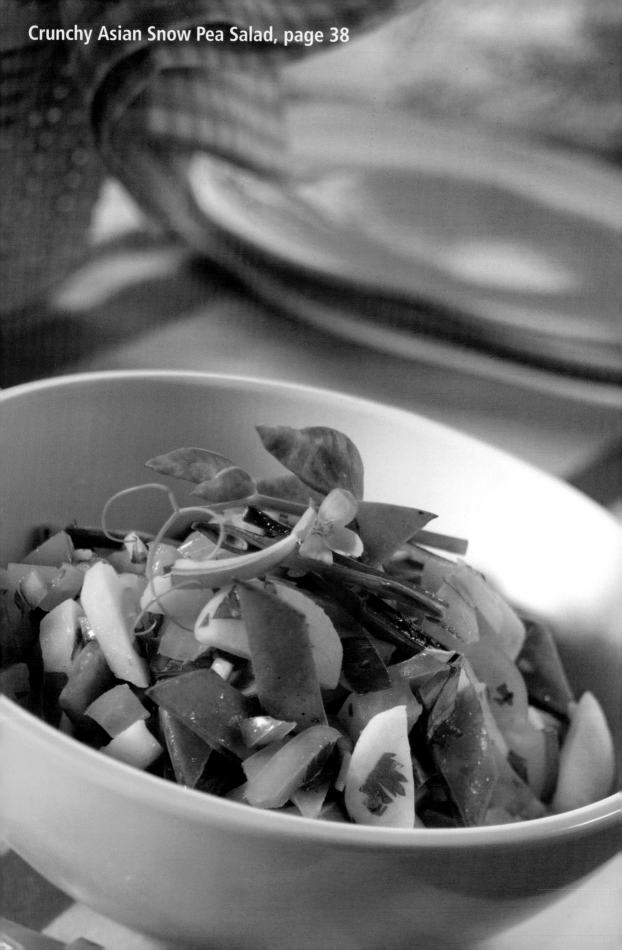

Crunchy Asian Snow Pea Salad, page 38

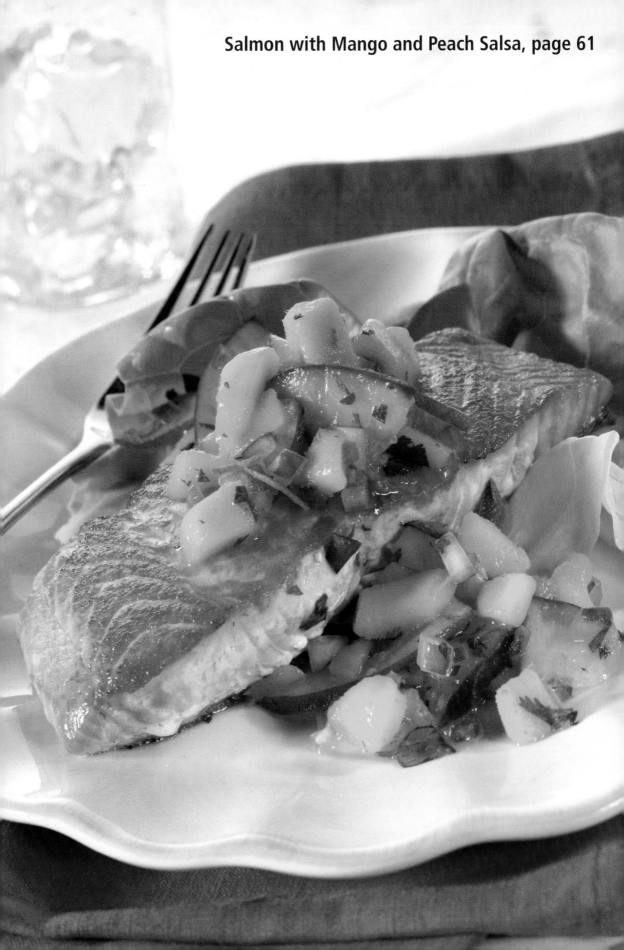

Salmon with Mango and Peach Salsa, page 61

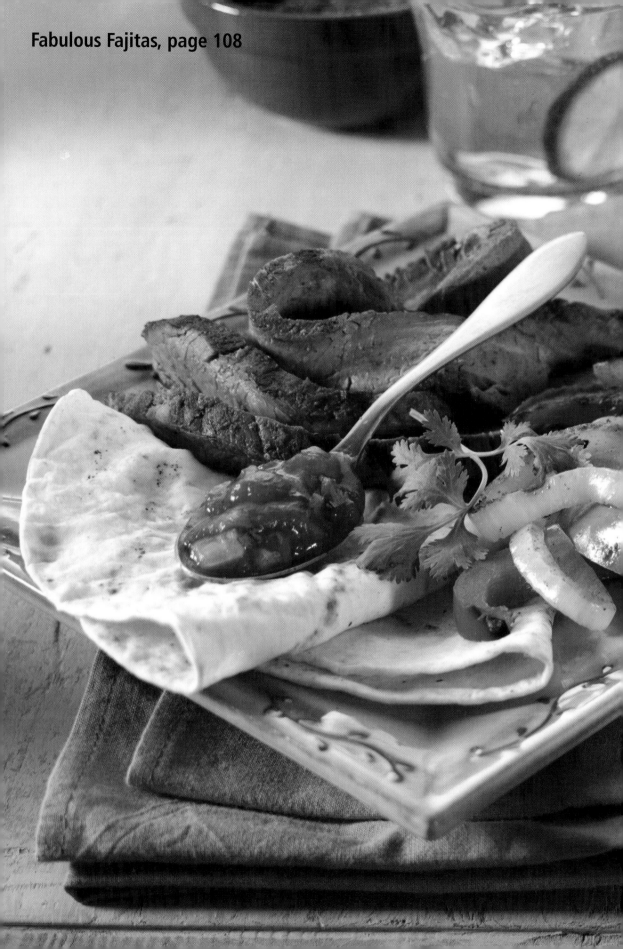

Fabulous Fajitas, page 108

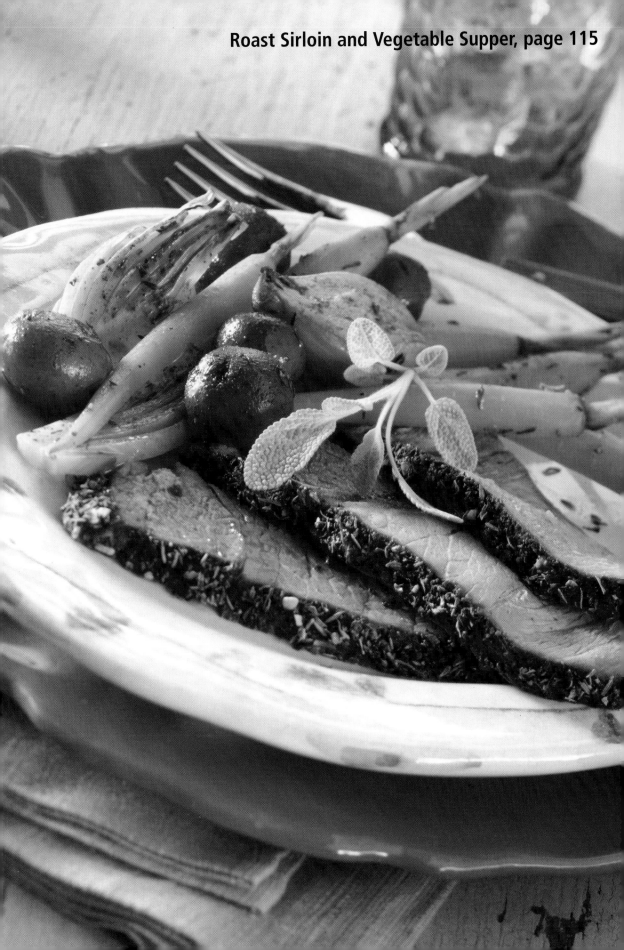

Roast Sirloin and Vegetable Supper, page 115

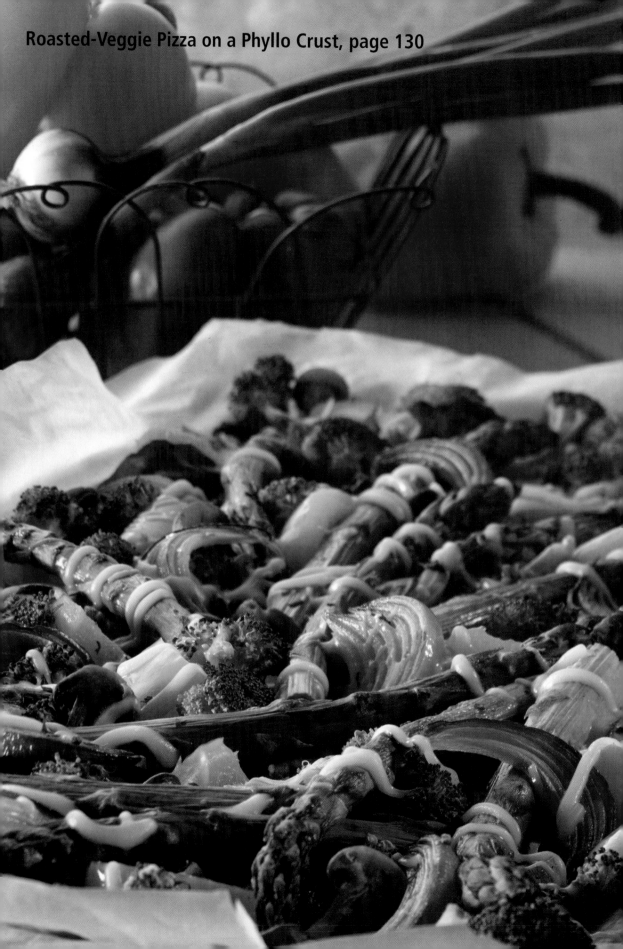

Roasted-Veggie Pizza on a Phyllo Crust, page 130

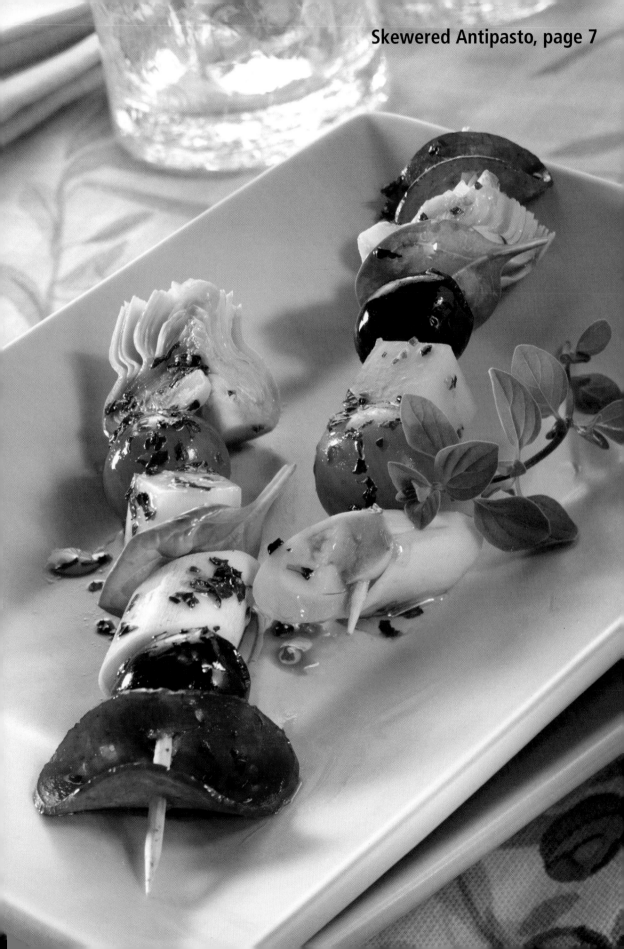

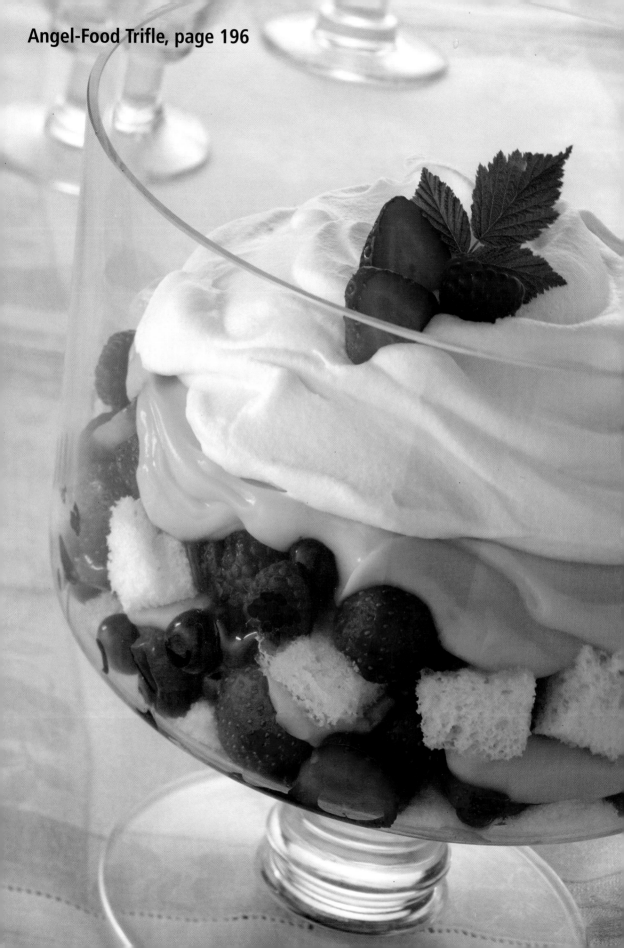

Angel-Food Trifle, page 196

Slow-Cooker Mediterranean Pot Roast

This simple, hearty dish is destined to become a family favorite.

Serves 8; 3 ounces cooked meat, 1/3 cup sauce, and 1 cup pasta per serving

- 3 medium garlic cloves, minced
- 2 teaspoons dried basil, crumbled
- 1 teaspoon dried oregano, crumbled
- 1/2 teaspoon salt
- 1/4 teaspoon crushed red pepper flakes
- 2 1/2-pound boneless top round steak or boneless chuck roast, all visible fat discarded
- 1 1/2 cups fat-free, low-sodium spaghetti sauce, such as tomato-basil, divided use
- 16 ounces dried whole-wheat spaghetti

1 Sprinkle the garlic, basil, oregano, salt, and red pepper flakes over both sides of the meat.

2 Pour 1 cup spaghetti sauce into a slow cooker. Place the meat on the sauce. Pour the remaining 1/2 cup sauce over the meat. Cook on low for 7 to 8 hours, or until the meat is fork tender. Transfer the meat to a cutting board. Cover loosely with aluminum foil. Spoon off and discard any fat from the sauce in the slow cooker.

3 About 12 minutes before serving time, prepare the spaghetti using the package directions, omitting the salt and oil. Drain well.

4 To serve, thinly slice the meat against the grain. Arrange the spaghetti on plates. Top with the meat. Ladle the sauce over all.

 COOK'S TIP
If the meat is too wide to fit into your slow cooker, cut the meat crosswise in half and stack it.

EXCHANGES

2 1/2 Starch
4 Very Lean Meat
1 Vegetable
1 Fat

Calories 407
   Calories from Fat 55
Total Fat..............................6 g
   Saturated Fat ....1.6 g
   Polyunsaturated Fat ....0.3 g
   Monounsaturated Fat .....2.1 g
Cholesterol ....80 mg
Sodium..........................233 mg
Total Carbohydrate.........46 g
   Dietary Fiber ....3 g
   Sugars ....5 g
Protein ....40 g

Mushroom-Smothered Cube Steak

This easy dish is somewhat like chicken-fried steak but with mushroom sauce instead of cream gravy.

Serves 4; 3 ounces steak and 1/3 cup mushroom sauce per serving

1/2 teaspoon salt
1/2 teaspoon pepper
4 cube steaks (about 4 ounces each), all visible fat discarded
2 tablespoons all-purpose flour
Vegetable oil spray
3 teaspoons canola oil, divided use
1/3 cup chopped shallots or sweet onion, such as Vidalia or Walla Walla
8 ounces button, cremini (brown), or mixed exotic mushrooms, sliced
2 medium garlic cloves, minced
1/2 cup fat-free, no-salt-added beef broth

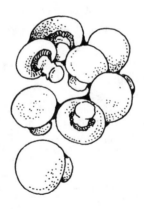

COOK'S TIP

Cube steaks are thin, boneless top sirloin or top or bottom round steaks that have been tenderized on a cubing machine.

1 Sprinkle the salt and pepper over the steaks. Put the flour in a shallow dish or bowl. Dredge the steaks in the flour, patting and turning until all the flour adheres to the steaks.

2 Heat a 12-inch nonstick skillet over medium-high heat. Remove from the heat and lightly spray with vegetable oil spray (being careful not to spray near a gas flame). Pour 2 teaspoons oil into the skillet and swirl to coat the bottom. When the oil is hot, cook the steaks, uncovered, for 3 minutes on each side, or until golden brown on the outside and pink in the center.

3 Place the steaks on an ovenproof platter. Cover with aluminum foil. Set the oven at 200°F. Put the platter in the oven.

4 Pour the remaining 1 teaspoon oil into the skillet. Swirl to coat. Reduce the heat to medium. Cook the shallots for 2 minutes, stirring occasionally.

5 Stir in the mushrooms and garlic. Cook for 5 minutes, stirring occasionally.

6 Stir in the broth. Reduce the heat and simmer, uncovered, until the sauce thickens, about 5 minutes.

7 To serve, put the steaks on plates. Spoon the mushroom sauce over the steaks.

EXCHANGES

3 Lean Meat
1/2 Carbohydrate

Calories 208
  Calories from Fat 79
Total Fat............................9 g
  Saturated Fat ....1.9 g
  Polyunsaturated Fat ....1.3 g
  Monounsaturated Fat .....4.3 g
Cholesterol ....64 mg
Sodium...........................344 mg
Total Carbohydrate...........9 g
  Dietary Fiber ....1 g
  Sugars ....2 g
Protein ....23 g

Fabulous Fajitas

A mixture of savory spices flavors this traditional Tex-Mex dish. (See photo insert.)

Serves 6; 1 fajita per serving

1 1/2	pounds flank steak, all visible fat and silver skin discarded (see Cook's Tip, page 104)
1/4	cup fresh lime juice
3	medium garlic cloves, minced
	Vegetable oil spray
2	teaspoons chili powder
2	teaspoons ground cumin
2	teaspoons ground coriander
1/4	teaspoon cayenne
2	large bell peppers (1 red and 1 green preferred), halved, stemmed, and seeded
2	1/4-inch-thick slices of a large onion (white or red)
6	8-inch fat-free flour tortillas
1/4	cup plus 2 tablespoons salsa
1/4	cup plus 2 tablespoons snipped fresh cilantro

COOK'S TIP

Make a double batch of the mixture of chili powder, cumin, coriander, and cayenne so you'll have extra to keep on hand. Stir some into canned refried black beans, or add some to tomato soup for a deep, rich flavor and color.

1 Put the steak in a shallow dish. Sprinkle with the lime juice and garlic. Cover the dish. Refrigerate for 30 minutes to 2 hours.

2 Lightly spray the grill rack or broiler pan and rack with vegetable oil spray. Preheat the grill on medium high or preheat the broiler.

3 In a small bowl, stir together the chili powder, cumin, coriander, and cayenne.

4 Remove the steak from the dish, leaving the garlic clinging to the steak. Put the steak on a flat surface. Discard the marinade. Lightly spray the bell pepper halves and onion slices with vegetable oil spray. Sprinkle the spice mixture evenly over both sides of the steak and vegetables. (The spray helps the seasoning adhere to the vegetables.) Put the steak and vegetables on the grill or on the rack of the broiler pan.

5 Grill or broil about 5 inches from the heat for 6 minutes. Turn over the steak and vegetables. Grill or broil for 5 to 6 minutes, or until the vegetables are tender and the steak is the desired doneness. Transfer to a cutting board. Lightly cover the steak with aluminum foil. Let stand for 5 minutes. Thinly slice the steak against the grain.

6 Meanwhile, cut the bell peppers into 1/4-inch strips. Separate the onion slices into rings. Using the package directions, warm the tortillas in a microwave oven.

7 To serve, place the steak and vegetables down the center of the tortillas. Top with the salsa and cilantro. Fold the sides of the tortillas over the filling. Place the fajitas on plates.

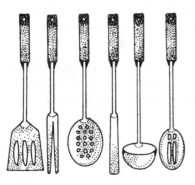

EXCHANGES

2 Starch
3 Lean Meat
2 Vegetable

Calories	348
Calories from Fat	79
Total Fat	9 g
Saturated Fat	3.5 g
Polyunsaturated Fat	0.6 g
Monounsaturated Fat	3.5 g
Cholesterol	54 mg
Sodium	510 mg
Total Carbohydrate	41 g
Dietary Fiber	5 g
Sugars	7 g
Protein	29 g

Spicy Orange Flank Steak

Tangy orange melds beautifully with robust garlic, spicy pepper flakes, and salty soy sauce in this grilled beef entrée.

Serves 4; 3 ounces steak per serving

---

    1 teaspoon grated orange zest
 1/4 cup fresh orange juice
    3 tablespoons light soy sauce
    3 medium garlic cloves, minced
 1/2 teaspoon crushed red pepper flakes
    1 pound flank steak, all visible fat and silver skin discarded
        (see Cook's Tip, page 104)
        Vegetable oil spray
    1 teaspoon grated orange zest

1 In a large airtight plastic bag or shallow dish, stir together 1 teaspoon orange zest, orange juice, soy sauce, garlic, and red pepper flakes. Add the steak, turning to coat. Seal the bag or cover the dish. Refrigerate for 30 minutes to 2 hours.

2 Lightly spray the grill rack with vegetable oil spray. Preheat the grill on medium high.

3 Meanwhile, drain the steak, pouring the marinade into a small saucepan. Bring the marinade to a boil over high heat. Boil for 5 minutes.

4 Place the steak on the grill. Brush with the marinade. Grill, covered, for 4 to 5 minutes on each side for medium-rare, or until desired doneness.

5 Place the steak on a cutting board. Lightly cover with aluminum foil. Let stand for 5 minutes. Thinly slice the steak against the grain.

6 To serve, place the steak on plates. Sprinkle with the remaining 1 teaspoon orange zest.

EXCHANGES

3 Lean Meat

Calories	183
Calories from Fat	73
Total Fat	8 g
Saturated Fat	3.5 g
Polyunsaturated Fat	0.3 g
Monounsaturated Fat	3.3 g
Cholesterol	54 mg
Sodium	360 mg
Total Carbohydrate	3 g
Dietary Fiber	0 g
Sugars	2 g
Protein	23 g

Tex-Mex Chili Bowl

This hearty chili pairs well with tossed green salad and corn bread.

Serves 4; 1 1/4 cups per serving

12 ounces boneless top round or lean chuck steak, all visible fat discarded
    Vegetable oil spray
1 medium onion, chopped
4 medium garlic cloves, minced
1 tablespoon chili powder
2 teaspoons ground cumin
1/4 teaspoon cayenne
1 cup fat-free, no-salt-added beef broth

14.5-ounce can no-salt-added diced tomatoes, undrained
2 15-ounce cans no-salt-added pinto or black beans, or one of each, rinsed and drained
1/2 cup salsa or picante sauce
1/4 cup crumbled queso fresco
1/4 cup snipped fresh cilantro
1/4 cup fat-free or light sour cream

1 Cut the steak into 3/4-inch cubes.

2 Heat a large saucepan over medium-high heat. Remove from the heat and lightly spray with vegetable oil spray (being careful not to spray near a gas flame). Cook the steak, onion, and garlic for 5 minutes, stirring frequently.

3 Stir in the chili powder, cumin, and cayenne. Cook for 1 minute, stirring frequently.

4 Pour in the broth. Increase the heat to high and bring to a boil. Reduce the heat and simmer, covered, for 1 hour, or until the steak is fork-tender, stirring once.

5 Stir in the tomatoes, beans, and salsa. Simmer, covered, for 10 minutes.

6 To serve, ladle the chili into bowls. Top with the cheese, cilantro, and sour cream.

Queso fresco is a tangy Mexican crumbling cheese. If it is not available, substitute farmer's cheese.

COOK'S TIP

EXCHANGES

2 1/2 Starch	3 Very Lean Meat
1/2 Fat	2 Vegetable

Calories 371
  Calories from Fat 53
Total Fat .... 6 g
  Saturated Fat .... 2.3 g
  Polyunsaturated Fat .... 0.8 g
  Monounsaturated Fat ..... 1.8 g
Cholesterol .... 54 mg
Sodium .... 234 mg
Total Carbohydrate .... 48 g
  Dietary Fiber .... 13 g
  Sugars .... 12 g
Protein .... 34 g

Slow-Cooker Swiss Steak

A slow cooker braises the meat to tender perfection in this traditional dish.

Serves 6; 3 ounces steak, 2/3 cup sauce, and scant 1 cup noodles per serving

2 tablespoons all-purpose flour
1 teaspoon dried basil, crumbled
1 teaspoon dried oregano, crumbled
1/2 teaspoon salt
1/2 teaspoon pepper
1 1/2 pounds boneless top round steak, all visible fat discarded
1 medium onion, thinly sliced
3 medium garlic cloves, thinly sliced

1 medium green bell pepper, cut into 3/4-inch pieces
1 1/2 cups fat-free, low-sodium spaghetti sauce, such as tomato-basil
8 ounces dried no-yolk egg noodles
1 teaspoon balsamic vinegar
2 tablespoons chopped fresh basil (optional)

1 In a small bowl, stir together the flour, dried basil, oregano, salt, and pepper.

2 Cut the beef into 6 pieces. Sprinkle half the flour mixture over one side of the beef. Using a meat tenderizer, meat mallet, or edge of a heavy saucer, pound the flour into the meat. Turn over. Repeat with the remaining flour mixture, pounding until all of it is absorbed into the meat.

3 Put the onion in the slow cooker. Put the meat on the onion. Sprinkle with the garlic, then with the bell pepper. Spoon the spaghetti sauce over all. Cook on low for 8 hours or on high for 4 hours, or until the meat is fork-tender.

4 About 15 minutes before serving time, prepare the noodles using the package directions, omitting the salt and oil.

5 To serve, spoon the noodles onto plates. Top with the meat. Stir the vinegar into the sauce. Spoon the sauce over all. Sprinkle with the fresh basil.

EXCHANGES

2 Starch
3 Very Lean Meat
2 Vegetable

Calories 322
Calories from Fat 36
Total Fat...........................4 g
Saturated Fat ....1.3 g
Polyunsaturated Fat ....0.3 g
Monounsaturated Fat .....1.5 g
Cholesterol ....60 mg
Sodium...........................256 mg
Total Carbohydrate.........38 g
Dietary Fiber ....3 g
Sugars ....8 g
Protein ....31 g

Both the pounding and the acid from the spaghetti sauce aid in tenderizing the beef.

COOK'S TIP

Grilled Sirloin with Tapenade

This entrée takes almost no time to prepare, looks appealing, and tastes wonderful.

Serves 6; 3 ounces meat and 1 heaping tablespoon tapenade per serving

SIRLOIN
Vegetable oil spray
1 1/2 pounds boneless top sirloin steak, about 1 inch thick, all visible fat discarded
1/2 tablespoon dried thyme, crumbled
4 medium garlic cloves, minced
1/2 teaspoon pepper
1/8 teaspoon salt

TAPENADE
1/4 cup chopped kalamata olives
3 tablespoons chopped pimiento-stuffed green olives
1 tablespoon Dijon mustard
1 tablespoon capers, rinsed and drained
1/2 teaspoon dried thyme, crumbled
1/2 medium garlic clove, minced

1 Lightly spray a grill rack with vegetable oil spray. Preheat the grill on medium high.

2 Lightly spray the steak with vegetable oil spray. Sprinkle with 1/2 tablespoon thyme, 4 cloves minced garlic, pepper, and salt, patting to coat.

3 Grill the steak, covered, for 10 minutes on each side for medium-rare, or until desired doneness. Place the steak on a cutting board. Lightly cover with aluminum foil. Let stand for 5 minutes. Thinly slice the steak against the grain.

4 Meanwhile, in a small bowl, stir together the tapenade ingredients.

5 To serve, place the steak on plates and top with the tapenade.

> **COOK'S TIP**
> *The word tapenade comes from tapeno, or capers. Originating in Provence, this multipurpose paste is made of capers, olives, garlic, and, usually, anchovies and olive oil. Try it on bruschetta, in salad dressing, or over steamed green beans. Make a double batch and keep the tapenade, covered and refrigerated, for up to one week.*

EXCHANGES

3 Lean Meat

Calories	158
Calories from Fat	56
Total Fat	6 g
Saturated Fat	2.2 g
Polyunsaturated Fat	0.3 g
Monounsaturated Fat	3.0 g
Cholesterol	65 mg
Sodium	341 mg
Total Carbohydrate	2 g
Dietary Fiber	0 g
Sugars	1 g
Protein	23 g

Sassy Beef and Onion Kebabs

These wonderfully spicy kebabs are perfect for the grilling season. Fresh corn on the cob, grilled at the same time, is a terrific accompaniment.

Serves 4; 1 kebab per serving

Vegetable oil spray	1/4 cup no-salt-added ketchup
1 pound boneless top sirloin steak, about 1 1/4 inches thick, all visible fat discarded	1 teaspoon red hot-pepper sauce
	3 medium garlic cloves, minced
	1 teaspoon dry mustard
1/4 cup beer (light, regular, or nonalcoholic)	1/2 teaspoon salt
	1 large onion

1 Lightly spray the grill rack with vegetable oil spray. Preheat the grill on medium high.

2 Meanwhile, cut the meat into 16 cubes. Put the meat in a large airtight plastic bag or shallow dish.

3 In a small nonmetallic bowl, stir together the remaining ingredients except the onion. Add to the meat, turning to coat. Seal the bag or cover the dish. Refrigerate for 30 minutes to 2 hours.

4 Drain the meat, pouring the marinade into a small saucepan. Bring the marinade to a boil over high heat. Boil for 5 minutes.

5 Meanwhile, cut the onion through the core into 16 wedges about 1/3 inch thick. Alternately thread the meat cubes and onion wedges on four metal skewers.

6 Place the kebabs on the grill. Brush with half the marinade.

7 Grill, covered, for 5 minutes. Turn over the kebabs. With a clean brush, brush with the remaining marinade. Grill, covered, for 5 to 8 minutes for medium-rare, or until desired doneness.

EXCHANGES

3 Lean Meat
1/2 Carbohydrate

Calories 191
Calories from Fat 47
Total Fat..............................5 g
Saturated Fat ....1.9 g
Polyunsaturated Fat ....0.2 g
Monounsaturated Fat .....2.1 g
Cholesterol ....65 mg
Sodium...........................352 mg
Total Carbohydrate.........11 g
Dietary Fiber ....1 g
Sugars ....8 g
Protein ....23 g

Cutting the onion through the core keeps the wedges attached by the root, making it easier to thread them onto the skewers.

COOK'S TIP

Roast Sirloin and Vegetable Supper

For carefree entertaining, try this easy one-dish meal. You can enjoy visiting with your company while dinner cooks. (See photo insert.)

Serves 8; 3 ounces meat and 1 cup vegetables per serving

Vegetable oil spray
2-pound boneless top sirloin steak, about 1 1/2 inches thick, all visible fat discarded
2 pounds red potatoes, cut into 1-inch pieces
8 ounces baby carrots
8 ounces medium shallots or large pearl onions, peeled
1 large fennel bulb, trimmed, or 1 large turnip, trimmed and peeled, cut into 1/2-inch-thick wedges

1 cup fat-free, no-salt-added beef broth
2 teaspoons dried thyme, crumbled
2 teaspoons paprika
1 teaspoon dried oregano, crumbled
3/4 teaspoon salt
1/2 teaspoon dried minced garlic or garlic powder
1/2 teaspoon dried sage, crumbled
1/2 teaspoon pepper

1 Preheat the oven to 350°F.

2 Spray a large, shallow roasting pan with vegetable oil spray. Put the steak in the center of the pan.

3 Arrange the potatoes, carrots, shallots, and fennel around the steak. Pour the broth over the vegetables.

4 In a small bowl, stir together the remaining ingredients. Sprinkle over the steak and vegetables.

5 Roast, uncovered, for 40 to 45 minutes, or until desired doneness. Put the steak on a cutting board. Lightly cover with aluminum foil. Let stand for 10 minutes.

6 Stir the vegetables. Test with a sharp knife for tenderness. If needed, roast, uncovered, for 5 to 10 minutes, or until tender.

7 To serve, thinly slice the steak against the grain. Place on plates. Arrange the vegetables around the steak. Spoon any pan juices over all.

EXCHANGES

1 1/2 Starch
2 Lean Meat
2 Vegetable

Calories	274
Calories from Fat	48
Total Fat	5 g
Saturated Fat	2.0 g
Polyunsaturated Fat	0.3 g
Monounsaturated Fat	2.1 g
Cholesterol	65 mg
Sodium	313 mg
Total Carbohydrate	31 g
Dietary Fiber	5 g
Sugars	5 g
Protein	26 g

Mexican-Style Stuffed Bell Peppers

In a new twist on stuffed bell peppers, black beans replace the rice and salsa replaces the tomato sauce.

Serves 4; 1 pepper per serving

- 4 large red or green bell peppers, or a combination
  Vegetable oil spray
- 1/2 cup chopped onion
- 3 medium garlic cloves, minced
- 8 ounces lean ground beef or lean ground turkey breast, skin removed before grinding
- 2 teaspoons chili powder
- 1 teaspoon ground cumin
- 1/4 teaspoon salt
- 3/4 cup salsa
- 1 cup drained canned no-salt-added black beans, rinsed
- 1/2 cup snipped fresh cilantro
- 1/2 cup reduced-fat shredded Mexican cheese blend
- 1/4 cup fat-free or light sour cream
- 2 tablespoons snipped fresh cilantro

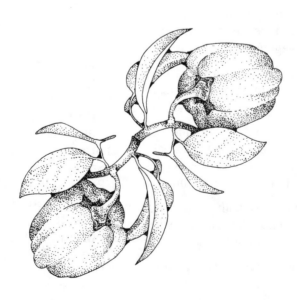

1 Preheat the oven to 375°F.

2 Cut the top 1/2 inch from each bell pepper. Discard the stems. Chop the bell pepper tops. Set aside. Discard the seeds and membrane from the bell pepper bottoms. Place the bell peppers with the cut side up on a paper towel in a microwave oven. Cook on 100 percent power (high) for 4 to 5 minutes, or until tender-crisp. Place the bell pepper bottoms with the cut side up in a 9-inch square baking dish or shallow casserole dish.

3 Meanwhile, heat a large nonstick skillet over medium heat. Remove from the heat and lightly spray with vegetable oil spray (being careful not to spray near a gas flame). Cook the chopped bell pepper, onion, and garlic for 5 minutes.

4 Add the meat. Cook for 5 minutes, stirring often to break up the meat. Pour off and discard the drippings.

5 Sprinkle the mixture with the chili powder, cumin, and salt. Cook for 1 minute. Stir in the salsa. Remove from the heat.

6 Stir in the beans and 1/2 cup cilantro. Spoon the meat mixture into the peppers. Cover the baking dish with aluminum foil.

7 Bake for 30 minutes, or until heated through. Remove from the oven. Sprinkle the cheese over the meat mixture. Let stand for 5 minutes, or until the cheese melts.

8 To serve, place the peppers on plates. Top with dollops of sour cream and a sprinkling of the remaining cilantro.

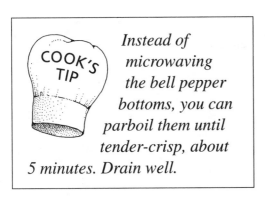

COOK'S TIP

Instead of microwaving the bell pepper bottoms, you can parboil them until tender-crisp, about 5 minutes. Drain well.

EXCHANGES

1 Starch
2 Lean Meat
3 Vegetable
1/2 Fat

Calories 276
　Calories from Fat 78
Total Fat............................9 g
　Saturated Fat ....3.4 g
　Polyunsaturated Fat ....0.7 g
　Monounsaturated Fat .....3.0 g
Cholesterol ....45 mg
Sodium..........................445 mg
Total Carbohydrate.........31 g
　Dietary Fiber ....7 g
　Sugars ....10 g
Protein ....22 g

Swedish Meatballs

Ground allspice gives these moist meatballs their remarkable flavor.

Serves 4; 5 meatballs, 1/3 cup sauce, and about 1 1/4 cups noodles per serving

---

- 2 slices rye bread (about 1 ounce each)
- 1 pound lean ground beef
- White of 1 large egg
- 1/4 cup fat-free milk
- 1/2 teaspoon ground allspice
- 1/8 teaspoon salt
- Vegetable oil spray
- 8 ounces dried no-yolk egg noodles
- 2 tablespoons all-purpose flour
- 1 cup fat-free, no-salt-added beef broth
- 1 cup fat-free or light sour cream
- 1 tablespoon low-sodium Worcestershire sauce
- 1/4 teaspoon pepper
- 2 tablespoons snipped fresh parsley or chopped fresh thyme

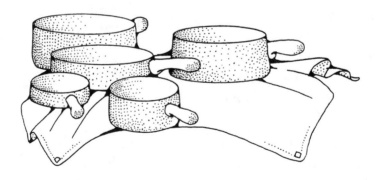

1 In a food processor or blender, process the bread into crumbs. Pour the crumbs into a medium bowl.

2 Combine the meat, egg white, milk, allspice, and salt with the crumbs. You'll get the best results by mixing with your hands, but you can use a spoon if you prefer. Shape the mixture into 20 meatballs, about 1 inch in diameter.

3 Heat a large, deep nonstick skillet over medium heat. Remove from the heat and lightly spray with vegetable oil spray (being careful not to spray near a gas flame). Cook the meatballs for 12 to 14 minutes, or until browned on all sides, turning occasionally. (The meatballs will not be done.) Place the meatballs on a plate. Set aside.

4 Meanwhile, prepare the noodles using the package directions, omitting the salt and oil. Drain well.

5 Put the flour in a small bowl. Gradually whisk in the broth. Put the mixture in the skillet and add the meatballs. Bring to a simmer over medium heat, whisking constantly. Reduce the heat and simmer for 1 minute, whisking occasionally.

6 Stir in the sour cream, Worcestershire sauce, and pepper. Return the meatballs to the skillet. Cook until the meatballs are no longer pink in the center, 6 to 8 minutes, stirring occasionally.

7 To serve, spoon the noodles onto plates. Spoon the meatballs and sauce over the noodles. Sprinkle with the parsley.

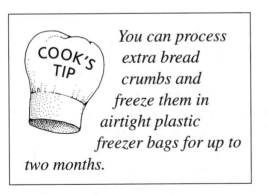

COOK'S TIP

You can process extra bread crumbs and freeze them in airtight plastic freezer bags for up to two months.

EXCHANGES

4 Starch
3 Lean Meat

Calories 511
Calories from Fat 94
Total Fat..........................10 g
Saturated Fat ....3.9 g
Polyunsaturated Fat ....0.6 g
Monounsaturated Fat .....4.3 g
Cholesterol ....73 mg
Sodium..........................418 mg
Total Carbohydrate.........63 g
Dietary Fiber ....4 g
Sugars ....9 g
Protein ....36 g

Grilled Meat Loaf

Grilling gives this tasty meat loaf added flavor and a pleasantly crisp crust.

Serves 4; 2 slices per serving

Vegetable oil spray
1 slice whole-wheat bread (about 1 ounce)
1 pound lean ground beef
1/3 cup minced onion
White of 1 large egg
1/4 teaspoon salt
1/4 teaspoon pepper
2 tablespoons no-salt-added ketchup
1 medium garlic clove, minced
2 tablespoons no-salt-added ketchup
1 tablespoon coarse-grain or Dijon mustard

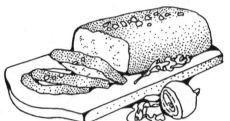

1 Lightly spray the grill rack with vegetable oil spray. Preheat the grill on medium high.

2 Meanwhile, in a food processor or blender, process the bread into crumbs. Pour the crumbs into a medium bowl.

3 Combine the meat, onion, egg white, salt, pepper, 2 tablespoons ketchup, and garlic with the crumbs. You'll get the best results by mixing with your hands, but you can use a spoon if you prefer. Shape the mixture into an oval patty 1 1/2 inches thick.

4 Grill the meat loaf, covered, for 10 minutes. Using two spatulas, carefully turn over the meat loaf.

5 Meanwhile, in a small bowl, stir together the remaining 2 tablespoons ketchup and the mustard. Spread over the top of the meat loaf.

6 Grill, covered, for 10 minutes, or until the meat loaf is no longer pink in the center.

7 To serve, put the meat loaf on a cutting board. Cut crosswise into 8 slices.

EXCHANGES

3 Lean Meat
1/2 Fat
1/2 Carbohydrate

Calories	229
Calories from Fat	88
Total Fat	10 g
Saturated Fat	3.8 g
Polyunsaturated Fat	0.4 g
Monounsaturated Fat	4.2 g
Cholesterol	69 mg
Sodium	357 mg
Total Carbohydrate	10 g
Dietary Fiber	1 g
Sugars	6 g
Protein	24 g

Southwestern Pork Tenderloin Skillet

This one-skillet dish showcases vibrant south-of-the-border flavors.

Serves 4; 2 pork medallions and 3/4 cup hominy mixture per serving

- 1 pound pork tenderloin, all visible fat discarded
- 2 teaspoons chili powder
- 1 teaspoon ground cumin
- 1/8 teaspoon cayenne
- 1 teaspoon canola oil
- 1 medium green bell pepper, cut into 1/2-inch squares
- 15-ounce can white hominy, rinsed and drained
- 1 cup frozen whole-kernel corn, thawed
- 1/2 cup salsa
- 2 tablespoons snipped fresh cilantro or green onions, thinly sliced (green part only)

1 Cut the tenderloin crosswise into 8 slices. Press down on each slice to flatten into medallions.

2 In a small bowl, stir together the chili powder, cumin, and cayenne. Set aside 1/2 teaspoon mixture. Rub the remaining mixture over both sides of the pork.

3 Heat a large nonstick skillet over medium-high heat. Pour in the oil and swirl to coat the bottom. Cook the pork for 3 minutes. Reduce the heat to medium. Turn over the pork and cook for 3 minutes. Transfer to a plate. Set aside.

4 Put the bell pepper in the skillet. Cook for 5 minutes, stirring occasionally.

5 Stir in the hominy, corn, salsa, and re-served spice mixture. Cook for 3 minutes, or until the bell pepper is tender.

6 Return the pork and any accumulated juices to the skillet. Cook for 4 minutes, or until the pork is no longer pink in the center, turning the pork once.

7 To serve, place the pork and the vegetable mixture on plates. Sprinkle with the cilantro.

EXCHANGES

1 Starch
3 Lean Meat
1 Vegetable

Calories	258
Calories from Fat	57
Total Fat	6 g
Saturated Fat	1.7 g
Polyunsaturated Fat	0.5 g
Monounsaturated Fat	2.5 g
Cholesterol	66 mg
Sodium	255 mg
Total Carbohydrate	24 g
Dietary Fiber	5 g
Sugars	5 g
Protein	26 g

Asian Barbecued Pork Tenderloin

Traditional Asian barbecued pork is slowly smoked and gets its bright red appearance from food coloring. This modern version gets its beautiful color and tangy flavor from a mixture of hickory barbecue sauce and Asian condiments.

Serves 4; 3 ounces pork per serving

MARINADE
2 tablespoons hickory barbecue sauce
1 tablespoon light soy sauce
1 tablespoon plain rice vinegar or cider vinegar
2 medium garlic cloves, minced
1 teaspoon minced peeled gingerroot
1/2 teaspoon Szechuan peppercorns, crushed, or 1/4 teaspoon crushed red pepper flakes

PORK
1 pound pork tenderloin, all visible fat discarded
Vegetable oil spray
1/4 cup water

1 In a large airtight plastic bag or glass baking dish, stir together the marinade ingredients. Add the pork and turn to coat. Seal the bag or cover the dish. Refrigerate for 30 minutes to 2 hours.

2 Lightly spray the grill rack or broiler pan and rack with vegetable oil spray. Preheat the grill on medium high or preheat the broiler.

3 Drain the tenderloin, pouring the marinade into a small saucepan. Pour in the water. Bring to a boil over high heat. Boil for 5 minutes.

4 Put the pork on the grill or broiler rack. Brush half the marinade over the pork. Grill the pork, covered, or broil 4 to 5 inches from the heat for 8 minutes. Turn over. Using a clean brush, brush with the remaining marinade. Grill, covered, or broil for 8 minutes. Turn over. Grill, covered, or broil for 2 to 4 minutes, or until the internal temperature measures 160°F or until desired doneness.

5 Put the pork on a cutting board. Lightly cover with aluminum foil. Let stand for 5 minutes.

6 To serve, cut crosswise into thin slices.

EXCHANGES

3 Lean Meat

Calories	148
Calories from Fat	37
Total Fat	4 g
Saturated Fat	1.4 g
Polyunsaturated Fat	0.4 g
Monounsaturated Fat	1.7 g
Cholesterol	66 mg
Sodium	251 mg
Total Carbohydrate	2 g
Dietary Fiber	0 g
Sugars	2 g
Protein	24 g

Spicy Pork Chops with Sweet Mango Sauce

Sweet mango pairs perfectly with spicy pork in this Jamaican-inspired dish.

Serves 4; 1 pork chop and 1/3 cup sauce per serving

Vegetable oil spray
1 teaspoon paprika
1 teaspoon dried thyme, crumbled
1/8 teaspoon ground allspice
1/8 teaspoon cayenne
1/2 teaspoon salt
4 boneless pork loin chops, 1/2 inch thick (about 4 ounces each), all visible fat discarded

1 tablespoon apricot all-fruit spread or pineapple preserves
1 medium mango, diced
2 tablespoons snipped fresh cilantro
1 tablespoon fresh lime juice

1. Lightly spray the grill rack with vegetable oil spray. Preheat the grill on medium high.

2. In a small bowl, stir together the paprika, thyme, allspice, and cayenne. Set aside 1/4 teaspoon mixture for the sauce.

3. Sprinkle the remaining spice mix and salt over the pork chops. Lightly spray with vegetable oil spray.

4. Grill the pork, covered, for 5 minutes on each side, or until no longer pink in the center.

5. Meanwhile, in a medium bowl, briskly stir the fruit spread until softened (a fork works well). Stir in the remaining ingredients, including the reserved spice mixture.

6. To serve, place the pork on plates. Top with the sauce.

 COOK'S TIP

If the preserves are very cold, soften them by microwaving at 100 percent power (high) for 15 seconds, or let them stand at room temperature for 5 minutes before stirring.

EXCHANGES

3 Lean Meat
1 Fruit

Calories	214
Calories from Fat	63
Total Fat	7 g
Saturated Fat	2.5 g
Polyunsaturated Fat	0.6 g
Monounsaturated Fat	3.0 g
Cholesterol	68 mg
Sodium	344 mg
Total Carbohydrate	13 g
Dietary Fiber	1 g
Sugars	11 g
Protein	24 g

Thyme-Scented Pork Chop and Bean Skillet

This pork-and-beans dish is ready in less than 30 minutes.

Serves 4; 3 pork strips and scant 1 cup beans per serving

- 1 teaspoon paprika
- 1 teaspoon dried thyme, crumbled
- 1/4 teaspoon pepper
- 1/4 teaspoon salt
- 3 boneless pork loin chops (about 4 ounces each), all visible fat discarded
  Vegetable oil spray
- 1/4 cup no-salt-added ketchup
- 2 tablespoons light brown sugar
- 1 tablespoon Dijon or spicy brown mustard
- 1 tablespoon low-sodium Worcestershire sauce
  15-ounce can no-salt-added kidney beans, rinsed and drained
  15-ounce can no-salt-added pinto beans, rinsed and drained

> **COOK'S TIP**
>
> The combination of ketchup, brown sugar, mustard, and Worcestershire sauce (ingredients you are likely to have) in this recipe makes a flavorful barbecue sauce. Prepare an extra batch to keep tightly covered in the refrigerator for up to one week. The sauce does not need to be cooked before you use it.

1 In a small bowl, stir together the paprika, thyme, pepper, and salt. Sprinkle over both sides of the pork chops.

2 Heat a large nonstick skillet over medium-high heat. Remove from the heat and lightly spray with vegetable oil spray (being careful not to spray near a gas flame). Cook the pork for 3 minutes on each side. Put on a cutting board. Cut each pork chop into 4 strips. Set aside.

3 Put the ketchup, brown sugar, mustard, and Worcestershire sauce in the skillet. Stir. Reduce the heat to low.

4 Stir in the kidney beans and pinto beans. Adjust the heat as needed and bring to a simmer. Simmer for 5 minutes.

5 Return the pork to the skillet. Increase the heat to medium. Cook for 2 minutes on each side, or until the pork is no longer pink in the center.

6 To serve, place the pork strips and beans on plates.

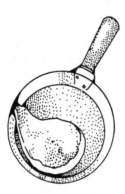

EXCHANGES

2 Starch
2 Lean Meat
1 Carbohydrate

Calories 335
  Calories from Fat 41
Total Fat..............................5 g
  Saturated Fat ....1.3 g
  Polyunsaturated Fat ....0.7 g
  Monounsaturated Fat .....1.7 g
Cholesterol ....49 mg
Sodium..........................289 mg
Total Carbohydrate........46 g
  Dietary Fiber ....11 g
  Sugars ....15 g
Protein ....28 g

Onion-Smothered Pork Chops

This hearty dish is ready in less than 30 minutes. It's perfect with mashed potatoes and steamed green beans.

Serves 4; 1 pork chop and about 1/4 cup onion per serving

1 teaspoon paprika
1 teaspoon dried sage or thyme, crumbled
1/4 teaspoon salt
1/4 teaspoon pepper
4 boneless center-cut pork chops, about 1/2 inch thick (about 4 ounces each), all visible fat discarded
Vegetable oil spray
2 large yellow or sweet onions, such as Vidalia or Walla Walla, thinly sliced
4 tablespoons low-fat, low-sodium chicken broth, divided use
1 tablespoon Dijon mustard (regular or hot)

1 Sprinkle the paprika, sage, salt, and pepper over the pork chops.

2 Heat a large nonstick skillet over medium heat. Remove from the heat and lightly spray with vegetable oil spray (being careful not to spray near a gas flame). Cook the pork for 4 minutes on each side. Put the pork on a plate. Set aside.

3 Separate the onion slices into rings. Put the onions in the skillet. Stir in 1 tablespoon broth. Cook, covered, for 5 minutes. Stir well. Cook, uncovered, for 5 minutes, or until the onions are golden brown, stirring once.

4 Stir in the remaining 3 tablespoons broth and mustard. Place the pork on the onions. Cook, uncovered, for 5 minutes, or until the onions are tender and the pork no longer is pink in the center.

5 To serve, place the pork on plates. Spoon the onions over the pork.

EXCHANGES

3 Lean Meat
2 Vegetable

Calories	214
Calories from Fat	65
Total Fat	7 g
Saturated Fat	2.5 g
Polyunsaturated Fat	0.7 g
Monounsaturated Fat	3.1 g
Cholesterol	69 mg
Sodium	296 mg
Total Carbohydrate	11 g
Dietary Fiber	2 g
Sugars	8 g
Protein	26 g

Ham and Broccoli Frittata

Serve this tasty egg dish with a tossed salad when you need to get supper on the table in a hurry.

Serves 4; 1 wedge per serving

Vegetable oil spray
2 cups frozen fat-free potatoes O'Brien, thawed
4 ounces small broccoli florets (about 3/4 cup)
Whites of 5 large eggs

Egg substitute equivalent to 1 egg, or 1 large egg
6 ounces lower-sodium, low-fat ham, cut into 1/4-inch cubes
1/4 cup fat-free milk
1/4 teaspoon pepper

1 Preheat the oven to 400°F.

2 Heat a 10-inch nonstick ovenproof skillet over medium heat. Remove from the heat and lightly spray with vegetable oil spray (being careful not to spray near a gas flame). Put the potatoes in the skillet. Lightly spray with vegetable oil spray. Cook for 4 to 5 minutes, or until golden brown, stirring occasionally.

3 Meanwhile, rinse the broccoli in cold water; drain but do not dry (some water droplets will cling to the broccoli). Put the broccoli in a microwave-safe bowl. Cook, covered, on 100 percent power (high) for 3 to 4 minutes, or until tender-crisp. Drain. Stir the broccoli into the potatoes.

4 In a medium bowl, whisk together the egg whites and egg substitute. Whisk in the ham, milk, and pepper. Pour the mixture over the potatoes and broccoli. Stir well.

5 Bake, uncovered, for 15 to 18 minutes, or until the eggs are set (they don't jiggle when gently shaken).

6 To serve, cut the frittata into wedges.

If your skillet is not oven-proof, wrap the handle in heavy aluminum foil before putting it in the oven.

COOK'S TIP

EXCHANGES

1/2 Starch	2 Very Lean Meat
1 Vegetable	

Calories 128
 Calories from Fat 9
Total Fat...............................1 g
 Saturated Fat ....0.3 g
 Polyunsaturated Fat ....0.2 g
 Monounsaturated Fat .....0.3 g
Cholesterol ....20 mg
Sodium...........................472 mg
Total Carbohydrate.........14 g
 Dietary Fiber ....2 g
 Sugars ....4 g
Protein ....15 g

Vegetarian
Entrées

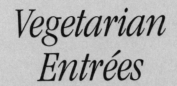

Roasted-Veggie Pizza on a Phyllo Crust

A colorful variety of fresh vegetables nests on paper-thin phyllo dough, then is topped with just enough cheese to delight. (See photo insert.)

Serves 8; 1/8 pizza per serving

	Vegetable oil spray (olive oil spray preferred)
12	ounces small broccoli florets (about 2 cups)
12	ounces asparagus, trimmed, cut into 2-inch pieces (about 2 cups)
3	ounces spinach leaves (about 2 cups, tightly packed)
6 to 7	ounces button mushrooms, thickly sliced (about 2 cups)
1	medium red, green, or yellow bell pepper, chopped
1/2	cup chopped red onion
1/4	teaspoon black pepper
6	sheets frozen phyllo dough, thawed
1/3	cup shredded part-skim mozzarella cheese
3	tablespoons shredded Parmesan cheese
1/4	teaspoon dried oregano or dried basil, crumbled
1/8	teaspoon crushed red pepper flakes

COOK'S TIP

Spelled phyllo, fillo, or filo, these fragile, paper-thin sheets of dough are usually found in the freezer section of the supermarket, near the piecrusts and puff pastry. Phyllo dough can also be found fresh at many Greek specialty food stores. It is made of flour and water, without any fat. When baked, phyllo will be flaky and crumbly.

1 Preheat the oven to 425°F.

2 Lightly spray a 15 × 10 × 1/2-inch nonstick baking pan with vegetable oil spray. Put the broccoli, asparagus, spinach, mushrooms, bell pepper, and onion in a single layer in the pan. Sprinkle with the black pepper. Lightly spray the vegetables with vegetable oil spray.

3 Roast the vegetables for 10 to 15 minutes, or until the onion is tender-crisp. Put the vegetables on a plate.

4 Wipe the pan with paper towels. Lightly spray the pan with vegetable oil spray.

5 Reduce the oven temperature to 400°F.

6 Working quickly so the phyllo won't dry out, stack the sheets on a flat surface. Remove 1 sheet from the stack and place it in the pan. Cover the remaining sheets with a damp cloth or damp paper towels. Lightly spray the sheet in the pan with vegetable oil spray. Repeat the layering and spraying process with the remaining phyllo.

7 To assemble the pizza, spread the roasted vegetables over the phyllo. Sprinkle with the remaining ingredients.

8 Bake for 10 to 15 minutes, or until the cheese has melted and the crust is golden brown around the edges.

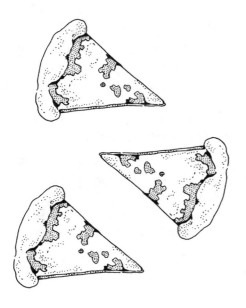

EXCHANGES

1/2 Starch
2 Vegetable
1/2 Fat

Calories 115
   Calories from Fat 26
Total Fat.............................3 g
   Saturated Fat ....0.9 g
   Polyunsaturated Fat ....0.5 g
   Monounsaturated Fat .....1.0 g
Cholesterol ....5 mg
Sodium..........................152 mg
Total Carbohydrate.........17 g
   Dietary Fiber ....3 g
   Sugars ....3 g
Protein ....6 g

Vegetable and Feta Focaccia

Pile cooked and raw veggies, lots of feta, and just a hint of rosemary on individual pizza dough rounds, then quickly bake them to perfection.

Serves 4; 1 pizza per serving

Vegetable oil spray (olive oil spray preferred)
1 small zucchini, thinly sliced (about 4 ounces)
1 small yellow summer squash, thinly sliced (about 4 ounces)
1 medium red bell pepper, thinly sliced
11-ounce tube refrigerated French bread dough
1/2 teaspoon dried rosemary, crushed
1/4 cup snipped fresh parsley
1 cup thinly sliced red onion
1/8 teaspoon crushed red pepper flakes
2 ounces crumbled feta cheese, rinsed and drained

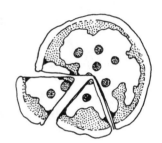

1 Preheat the oven to 350°F.

2 Heat a 12-inch nonstick skillet over medium-high heat. Remove from the heat and lightly spray with vegetable oil spray (being careful not to spray near a gas flame). Cook the zucchini, yellow squash, and bell pepper for 4 minutes, or until the zucchini is tender-crisp, stirring frequently.

3 Meanwhile, unroll the dough on a flat work surface. The pizza dough does not have to be perfectly shaped; a rustic look is fine. Cut into four rectangles. Place on a nonstick baking sheet. Lightly spray the dough with vegetable oil spray.

4 To assemble the pizzas, sprinkle each piece with the rosemary, parsley, and onion (in that order). Spoon the cooked vegetables over each piece. Sprinkle with the red pepper flakes and feta.

5 Bake for 20 minutes, or until the edges of the crust are golden.

EXCHANGES

2 Starch
1 Fat
2 Vegetable

Calories	270
Calories from Fat	52
Total Fat	6 g
Saturated Fat	2.8 g
Polyunsaturated Fat	0.5 g
Monounsaturated Fat	1.5 g
Cholesterol	13 mg
Sodium	628 mg
Total Carbohydrate	43 g
Dietary Fiber	3 g
Sugars	9 g
Protein	10 g

Six-Ingredient Lasagna

This six-ingredient one-dish meal will please the whole family.

Serves 6; 4 × 2 1/2-inch or 4 1/2 × 3-inch piece per serving

25.5-ounce jar fat-free, low-sodium pasta or spaghetti sauce, such as roasted garlic or tomato-basil
1/4 teaspoon crushed red pepper flakes (optional)
15-ounce container fat-free or low-fat ricotta cheese
2 tablespoons chopped fresh basil leaves
4 dried oven-ready or regular 10 × 2 1/2-inch lasagna noodles
1 1/2 cups shredded part-skim mozzarella cheese, divided use
3 tablespoons chopped fresh basil leaves

1 Preheat the oven to 375°F.

2 In a large skillet, stir together the pasta sauce and red pepper flakes. Bring to a simmer over medium-high heat. Reduce the heat and simmer, uncovered, for 5 minutes, stirring occasionally.

3 In a medium bowl, stir together the ricotta cheese and 2 tablespoons basil.

4 In an 8- or 9-inch square baking pan, layer 3/4 cup sauce, 2 noodles, half the ricotta mixture, half the mozzarella, 3/4 cup sauce, 2 noodles, remaining ricotta mixture, and remaining sauce. Cover with aluminum foil.

5 Bake for 40 minutes. Top with the remaining mozzarella. Bake, uncovered, for 15 minutes, or until bubbly. Let stand at room temperature for 5 minutes before cutting into 6 pieces.

EXCHANGES

1 Starch
2 Very Lean Meat
2 Lean Meat
2 Vegetable
1/2 Fat

Calories 218
  Calories from Fat 43
Total Fat...............................5 g
  Saturated Fat ....3.0 g
  Polyunsaturated Fat ....0.2 g
  Monounsaturated Fat .....1.3 g
Cholesterol ....39 mg
Sodium...........................209 mg
Total Carbohydrate.........24 g
  Dietary Fiber ....1 g
  Sugars ....10 g
Protein ....20 g

Eggplant Ricotta Lasagna

This is a great make-ahead entrée. In fact, it's even better the next day.

Serves 4; 4-inch square per serving

Vegetable oil spray
4 1/2 dried 10 × 2 1/2-inch lasagna noodles
8 ounces chopped unpeeled eggplant (about 3 cups)
1 small zucchini, sliced (about 4 ounces)
1 large onion, chopped
2 medium garlic cloves, minced
2 cups fat-free, low-sodium spaghetti sauce
1 tablespoon dried basil, crumbled
1/2 tablespoon dried oregano, crumbled
1 cup fat-free or low-fat ricotta cheese
1/2 teaspoon salt, divided use
1/2 cup shredded part-skim mozzarella cheese
1/4 cup shredded Parmesan cheese

1 Preheat the oven to 350°F. Lightly spray an 8-inch square baking pan with vegetable oil spray.

2 Prepare the noodles using the package directions, omitting the salt and oil. Drain well.

3 Meanwhile, heat a 12-inch nonstick skillet over medium-high heat. Remove from the heat and lightly spray with vegetable oil spray (being careful not to spray near a gas flame). Put the eggplant, zucchini, onion, and garlic in the skillet. Lightly spray with vegetable oil spray. Cook for 6 to 7 minutes, or until the zucchini is just tender, stirring frequently. Remove from the heat.

4 In a small bowl, stir together the spaghetti sauce, basil, and oregano.

5 To assemble, cut the 4 whole noodles in half crosswise. Place 3 noodle halves in one layer in the pan. Spread 2/3 cup spaghetti sauce mixture over the noodles. Using a teaspoon, dot 1/2 cup ricotta cheese over the sauce. Spoon 1 cup cooked vegetables evenly over all. Sprinkle with 1/4 teaspoon salt. Repeat. Top with the remaining 3 noodle halves. Spoon 2/3 cup sauce over all. Sprinkle with the mozzarella.

6 Bake, uncovered, for 30 minutes. Sprinkle with the Parmesan. Let stand for 15 minutes before cutting.

EXCHANGES

1 1/2 Starch	1 Lean Meat
4 Vegetable	

Calories 281
Calories from Fat 43
Total Fat..............................5 g
Saturated Fat ....2.6 g
Polyunsaturated Fat ....0.5 g
Monounsaturated Fat .....1.3 g
Cholesterol ....33 mg
Sodium..............................477 mg
Total Carbohydrate.........41 g
Dietary Fiber ....4 g
Sugars ....17 g
Protein ....20 g

White Bean and Brown Rice Casserole with Mozzarella

Rich-tasting, creamy melted cheese topped with a sprinkling of mild green chilies covers a hearty casserole.

Serves 4; 1 1/2 cups per serving

1 cup uncooked brown rice
Vegetable oil spray
1 1/2 15-ounce cans navy beans, rinsed and drained
3/4 cup finely chopped green onions (green and white parts)
3 tablespoons fresh lime juice
1 tablespoon ground cumin
1/8 to 1/4 teaspoon cayenne
3/8 teaspoon salt
1 1/4 cups shredded part-skim mozzarella cheese
6 ounces canned chopped green chilies, rinsed and drained

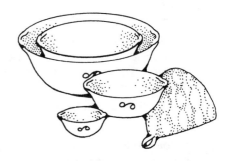

1 Prepare the rice using the package directions, omitting the salt and margarine.

2 Meanwhile, preheat the oven to 400°F.

3 Lightly spray an 11 × 7 × 2-inch glass baking dish with vegetable oil spray. In the baking dish, stir together the cooked rice, beans, green onions, lime juice, cumin, cayenne, and salt. Spread evenly. Sprinkle with the cheese.

4 Bake for 20 minutes, or until the cheese melts.

5 To serve, spoon the mixture onto each plate. Sprinkle with the green chilies.

EXCHANGES

4 1/2 Starch
1 Medium-Fat Meat

Calories	436
Calories from Fat	72
Total Fat	8 g
Saturated Fat	4.0 g
Polyunsaturated Fat	1.0 g
Monounsaturated Fat	2.5 g
Cholesterol	20 mg
Sodium	501 mg
Total Carbohydrate	69 g
Dietary Fiber	10 g
Sugars	4 g
Protein	22 g

Mexican Yellow Rice and Black Beans

So much color in one simple dish! Black beans nest on a bed of turmeric-colored rice, with orange Cheddar and dark green cilantro sprinkled over all.

Serves 4; 1 1/2 cups per serving

3/4 cup uncooked rice
1/2 teaspoon ground turmeric
 Vegetable oil spray (olive oil spray preferred)
1 large onion, chopped
1 large Anaheim pepper, seeds and ribs discarded, chopped (about 5 ounces), or 1 medium green bell pepper, chopped
1 medium red bell pepper, chopped

1/8 teaspoon crushed red pepper flakes
 15-ounce can no-salt-added black beans, rinsed and drained
1/2 teaspoon ground cumin
1/2 teaspoon salt
1 tablespoon olive oil
2 ounces fat-free or reduced-fat sharp Cheddar cheese, shredded
1/4 cup snipped fresh cilantro
2 medium limes, quartered

1 Prepare the rice using the package directions, adding the turmeric and omitting the salt and margarine.

2 Meanwhile, heat a 12-inch nonstick skillet over medium-high heat. Remove from the heat and lightly spray with vegetable oil spray (being careful not to spray near a gas flame). Put the onion, Anaheim pepper, bell pepper, and red pepper flakes in the skillet. Lightly spray with vegetable oil spray. Cook for 4 minutes, or until beginning to lightly brown on the edges, stirring frequently. Remove from the heat.

3 Stir in the beans, cumin, and salt. Let stand, covered, for 5 minutes. Stir in the oil.

4 To serve, spoon the rice onto a platter. Top with the bean mixture. Sprinkle with the cheese and cilantro. Serve with lime to squeeze over all.

EXCHANGES

3 Starch	2 Vegetable
1/2 Fat	

Calories 316
 Calories from Fat 38
Total Fat..............................4 g
 Saturated Fat ....0.5 g
 Polyunsaturated Fat ....0.6 g
 Monounsaturated Fat .....2.6 g
Cholesterol ....2 mg
Sodium..............................402 mg
Total Carbohydrate.........57 g
 Dietary Fiber ....6 g
 Sugars ....9 g
Protein ....14 g

> COOK'S TIP
>
> *Don't underestimate the power of the lime. It gives great flavor and a lot of zing to this dish, which can also be used to serve 12 as a side dish.*

Red Beans and Brown Rice

In Louisiana, this down-home food was customarily prepared on wash day, an all-day event before washing machines and dryers. That meant wash day was a good time to set a slow-cooking pot of dried beans on the stove to simmer. By the time the clothes were washed and dried, the beans were cooked to tenderness. This recipe calls for canned beans, so you can enjoy it any day of the week, wash day or not!

Serves 4; 1 1/2 cups per serving

1/2 tablespoon olive oil
1 medium onion, chopped
1 medium green bell pepper, chopped
1 medium red bell pepper, chopped
1/2 medium carrot, finely chopped
2 medium garlic cloves, minced
1/2 cup uncooked brown rice
1 teaspoon dried thyme, crumbled
1 teaspoon ground cumin

1/4 teaspoon crushed red pepper flakes
1/4 teaspoon salt
14.5-ounce can no-salt-added diced tomatoes, undrained
8-ounce can no-salt-added tomato sauce
1 cup water
15-ounce can no-salt-added kidney beans, rinsed and drained

1 Heat a large nonstick skillet over medium-high heat. Pour the oil into the pan and swirl to coat the bottom. Cook the onion, bell peppers, carrot, and garlic for 3 to 4 minutes, or until the onion is tender, stirring occasionally.

2 Stir in the rice, thyme, cumin, red pepper flakes, and salt. Cook for 1 minute, stirring to coat the rice.

3 Stir in the undrained tomatoes, tomato sauce, and water. Increase the heat to high and bring to a boil. Reduce the heat and simmer, covered, for 50 minutes, or until the rice is almost tender.

4 Stir in the beans. Cook for 10 to 15 minutes, or until the rice is tender and most of the liquid is absorbed.

EXCHANGES

2 Starch
4 Vegetable
1/2 Fat

Calories 265
 Calories from Fat 29
Total Fat..............................3 g
 Saturated Fat ....0.4 g
 Polyunsaturated Fat ....0.8 g
 Monounsaturated Fat .....1.6 g
Cholesterol ....0 mg
Sodium..........................213 mg
Total Carbohydrate.........51 g
 Dietary Fiber ....11 g
 Sugars ....13 g
Protein ....10 g

Stir-Fry Vegetables and Brown Rice

Broccoli stir-fry vegetables combine with asparagus and brown rice to make a dish that is as delicious as it is nutritious.

Serves 4; 1 cup vegetables and 1/2 cup rice per serving

1/2 cup uncooked brown rice
2 teaspoons canola oil
1/4 cup sliced green onions (green and white parts)
1 medium garlic clove, minced
1 teaspoon minced peeled gingerroot
1/4 teaspoon crushed red pepper flakes
4 ounces asparagus, trimmed, cut on the diagonal into 1-inch pieces

16-ounce package frozen unseasoned broccoli stir-fry vegetables or combination of your choice
1/3 cup reduced-sodium vegetable broth
1 tablespoon light soy sauce
1 tablespoon plain rice vinegar or white wine vinegar
2 teaspoons cornstarch
3 tablespoons water
2 tablespoons chopped green onions (green part only)

1 Prepare the rice using the package directions, omitting the salt and margarine.

2 About 10 minutes before the rice is ready, heat a wok or large nonstick skillet over medium heat. Pour in the oil and swirl to coat the bottom. Cook 1/4 cup green onions, garlic, gingerroot, and red pepper flakes for 1 minute, stirring occasionally.

3 Increase the heat to medium high. Stir in the asparagus. Cook for 1 minute, stirring frequently.

4 Stir in the stir-fry vegetables. Cook for 4 to 6 minutes, or until tender-crisp, stirring constantly.

5 Stir in the broth, soy sauce, and vinegar. Cook for 1 minute, stirring occasionally.

6 Put the cornstarch in a cup. Add the water, stirring to dissolve. Stir into the vegetable mixture. Cook for 1 minute, or until thickened, stirring frequently.

7 To serve, spread the rice on a platter. Spoon the vegetable mixture over the rice. Sprinkle with the chopped green onions.

EXCHANGES

1 Starch	2 Vegetable
1/2 Fat	

Calories	163
Calories from Fat	27
Total Fat	3 g
Saturated Fat	0.3 g
Polyunsaturated Fat	0.9 g
Monounsaturated Fat	1.6 g
Cholesterol	0 mg
Sodium	210 mg
Total Carbohydrate	28 g
Dietary Fiber	4 g
Sugars	5 g
Protein	4 g

Spinach, Artichoke, and Mushroom Toss

To create a sensation at your next dinner party or to step up a midweek meal, try this easy, flavorful skillet dish. It's loaded with vegetables, topped with feta, and served over hot, fluffy brown rice.

Serves 4; 1 cup vegetable mixture and 1/2 cup rice per serving

3/4 cup uncooked brown rice
    Vegetable oil spray
1 large onion, chopped
8 ounces sliced button mushrooms
2 medium garlic cloves, minced
1 teaspoon dried oregano, crumbled
1/8 teaspoon crushed red pepper flakes
2 ounces coarsely chopped fresh spinach leaves (about 2 cups)

14-ounce can quartered artichoke hearts, rinsed, drained, and coarsely chopped
1/2 cup chopped roasted red bell peppers, rinsed and drained if bottled
4 ounces feta cheese, crumbled
1/4 cup snipped fresh parsley

1   In a small saucepan, prepare the rice using the package directions, omitting the salt and margarine.

2   Meanwhile, heat a 12-inch nonstick skillet over medium-high heat. Remove from the heat and lightly spray with vegetable oil spray (being careful not to spray near a gas flame). Cook the onion for 4 minutes, or until beginning to brown slightly on the edges, stirring frequently.

3   Stir in the mushrooms, garlic, oregano, and red pepper flakes. Lightly spray with vegetable oil spray. Cook for 6 minutes, or until the mushrooms begin to lightly brown, stirring frequently.

4   Stir in the spinach, artichokes, and roasted peppers. Cook for 1 minute, or until the mixture is hot and the spinach begins to release moisture, stirring gently. Remove from the heat.

5   To serve, spoon the rice onto a platter. Top with the vegetable mixture. Sprinkle with the feta, parsley, and salt.

EXCHANGES

2 Starch   3 Vegetable
1 Fat

Calories 274
   Calories from Fat 71
Total Fat..............................8 g
   Saturated Fat ....4.4 g
   Polyunsaturated Fat ....0.8 g
   Monounsaturated Fat .....1.7 g
Cholesterol ....25 mg
Sodium..........................579 mg
Total Carbohydrate.........42 g
   Dietary Fiber ....5 g
   Sugars ....8 g
Protein ....11 g

Squash Stuffed with Brown Rice and Roasted Peppers

Brimming with flavor, these squash halves are piled high with brown rice and veggies and smothered in cheese.

Serves 4; 2 squash halves and 1 cup rice mixture per serving

	Vegetable oil spray
2/3	cup uncooked brown rice
4	medium yellow summer squash or zucchini, halved lengthwise
1 1/2	large onions, chopped
1	tablespoon dried basil, crumbled
1	medium garlic clove, minced
1/4	teaspoon crushed red pepper flakes
8	ounces roasted red bell peppers, rinsed and drained if bottled, chopped (about 1 cup)
1/2	cup snipped fresh parsley
1/4	teaspoon salt
1	cup shredded reduced-fat sharp Cheddar cheese

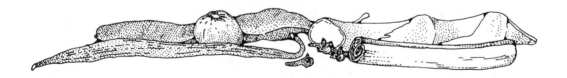

1 Preheat the oven to 350°F. Lightly spray a 13 × 9 × 2-inch baking pan with vegetable oil spray.

2 Prepare the rice using the package directions, omitting the salt and margarine.

3 Meanwhile, using a measuring teaspoon or melon ball scoop, scrape and reserve the seeds and most of the flesh from the squash, leaving the shells intact. Place the squash shells with the cut side up in the baking pan. Set aside. Coarsely chop the squash flesh and seeds.

4 Heat a 12-inch nonstick skillet over medium-high heat. Remove from the heat and lightly spray with vegetable oil spray (being careful not to spray near a gas flame). Cook the onions for 4 minutes, or until tender, stirring frequently.

5 Stir the chopped squash, basil, garlic, and red pepper flakes into the skillet. Cook for 5 minutes, or until the squash is tender, stirring frequently. Remove from the heat. Stir in the rice, red bell peppers, parsley, and salt.

6 Spoon about 1/2 cup rice mixture into each of the squash halves, pressing down firmly with a spoon or your fingertips. Cover the pan with aluminum foil.

7 Bake for 30 minutes, or until the squash shells are tender. Sprinkle with the cheese. Bake for 5 minutes, or until the cheese has melted. Let stand for 5 minutes.

EXCHANGES

2 Starch
3 Vegetable
1 Fat

Calories	274
Calories from Fat	70
Total Fat	8 g
Saturated Fat	3.7 g
Polyunsaturated Fat	0.8 g
Monounsaturated Fat	2.2 g
Cholesterol	20 mg
Sodium	477 mg
Total Carbohydrate	46 g
Dietary Fiber	8 g
Sugars	13 g
Protein	14 g

Lentils with Brown Rice and Mushrooms

Whether you serve this as a vegetarian entrée or a delicious side dish with one of the meat or poultry dishes in this cookbook, you're sure to enjoy the combination of flavors and textures it provides.

Serves 4; 1 1/2 cups per serving

3 cups reduced-sodium vegetable broth or water
3/4 cup dried lentils, sorted for stones and shriveled lentils and rinsed
1/2 cup uncooked brown rice
2 teaspoons olive oil
1 large onion, chopped
2 cups chopped button mushrooms
2 medium garlic cloves, minced
1 teaspoon ground cumin
1/4 teaspoon crushed red pepper flakes
1 teaspoon grated orange zest
3 tablespoons fresh orange juice
1 tablespoon light soy sauce
3 tablespoons minced fresh cilantro or parsley

> **COOK'S TIP**
>
> *The cooking time for lentils varies from about 25 minutes for red lentils to about 45 minutes for most other varieties. When lentils are done, they should be tender but hold their shape and not be mushy. When lentils are a little more than halfway through the expected cooking time, taste a couple, then repeat every 5 minutes until they are as tender as you want.*

1 In a medium saucepan, bring the broth to a boil over high heat. Stir in the lentils and return to a boil. Reduce the heat and simmer, covered, for 10 minutes.

2 Stir in the rice. Simmer, covered, for 25 to 30 minutes, or until the lentils and rice are tender and almost all the liquid is absorbed.

3 Meanwhile, heat a medium nonstick skillet over medium-low heat. Pour in the oil and swirl to coat the bottom. Cook the onion, mushrooms, and garlic for 10 to 12 minutes, or until the onion is very soft and nicely browned, stirring occasionally.

4 Stir in the cumin, red pepper flakes, and orange zest. Cook for 1 minute, stirring frequently.

5 Stir in the orange juice and soy sauce. Cook for 1 minute.

6 Stir the onion mixture and cilantro into the lentils and rice. Cook for 1 minute, or until hot.

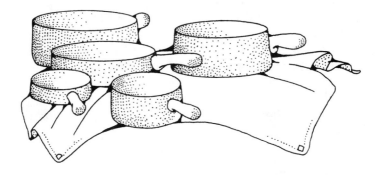

EXCHANGES

2 1/2 Starch
1 Vegetable
1/2 Fat

Calories 260
   Calories from Fat 33
Total Fat...........................4 g
   Saturated Fat ....0.5 g
   Polyunsaturated Fat ....0.7 g
   Monounsaturated Fat .....2.0 g
Cholesterol ....0 mg
Sodium..........................421 mg
Total Carbohydrate.........46 g
   Dietary Fiber ....9 g
   Sugars ....8 g
Protein ....12 g

Vegetable Chili with Mixed Beans

Cumin, paprika, green chilies, and chili powder season this meatless version of a favorite dish. Try it over brown rice, barley, or even couscous to soak up the wonderful liquid.

Serves 4; 2 cups per serving

2 teaspoons canola oil
1 large onion, chopped
1 medium red, green, or yellow bell pepper, chopped
1 medium rib of celery, chopped
1 medium carrot, chopped
3 medium garlic cloves, minced
1/4 ounce dried oyster or porcini mushrooms, snipped
4 ounces button or cremini (brown) mushrooms, chopped
1/4 cup canned green chilies, rinsed and drained
1 teaspoon chili powder
1/2 teaspoon ground cumin

1/2 teaspoon paprika
14.5-ounce can no-salt-added diced tomatoes, undrained
1 1/2 cups low-sodium vegetable broth or water
15-ounce can no-salt-added kidney beans, rinsed and drained
15-ounce can cannellini beans, rinsed and drained
8-ounce can no-salt-added tomato sauce
3 tablespoons snipped fresh cilantro or Italian (flat-leaf) parsley

EXCHANGES

2 1/2 Starch
4 Vegetable
1/2 Fat

Calories	302
Calories from Fat	33
Total Fat	4 g
Saturated Fat	0.2 g
Polyunsaturated Fat	1.4 g
Monounsaturated Fat	1.5 g
Cholesterol	0 mg
Sodium	336 mg
Total Carbohydrate	55 g
Dietary Fiber	16 g
Sugars	15 g
Protein	15 g

1 Heat a large nonstick saucepan over medium heat. Pour the oil into the pan and swirl to coat the bottom. Cook the onion, bell pepper, celery, and carrot for 8 to 10 minutes, or until the carrot is tender, stirring frequently. Increase the heat to medium high.

2 Stir in the garlic, dried mushrooms, and fresh mushrooms. Cook for 2 to 4 minutes, or until the fresh mushrooms begin to soften.

3 Stir in the chilies, chili powder, cumin, and paprika. Cook for 1 minute.

4 Stir in the remaining ingredients except the cilantro. Bring to a boil. Reduce the heat and simmer, partially covered, for 30 minutes.

5 Stir in the cilantro and cook for 1 minute.

Bean and Cheese Tostadas

A combination of giant nachos and tossed salad, these yummy (but messy) tostadas require knives and forks.

Serves 4; 1 tortilla, 1/4 cup bean mixture, and 3/4 cup lettuce mixture per serving

15-ounce can no-salt-added pinto beans, rinsed and drained
1/4 cup water
1 medium garlic clove, minced
2 teaspoons chili powder
1 teaspoon ground cumin
1/4 teaspoon red hot-pepper sauce
4 6-inch corn tortillas
1/2 cup shredded reduced-fat sharp Cheddar cheese

2 cups shredded lettuce
4 ounces grape tomatoes or cherry tomatoes, quartered (about 1/2 cup)
1/3 cup finely chopped red onion
1/4 cup snipped fresh cilantro
1 tablespoon fresh lime juice
2 teaspoons olive oil
1/4 teaspoon salt

1 Preheat the oven to 350°F.

2 In a food processor or blender, process the beans, water, garlic, chili powder, cumin, and hot-pepper sauce until smooth.

3 Put the tortillas on a baking sheet. Spread the bean mixture on each tortilla. Sprinkle with the cheese.

4 Bake for 10 minutes, or until the cheese has melted and the bean mixture is hot.

5 Meanwhile, in a medium bowl, gently toss the remaining ingredients.

6 When the tortillas are ready, spoon the lettuce mixture on each. Serve immediately.

EXCHANGES

2 Starch
1 Vegetable
1 Fat

Calories 216
  Calories from Fat 60
Total Fat............................7 g
  Saturated Fat ....2.2 g
  Polyunsaturated Fat ....0.9 g
  Monounsaturated Fat .....2.9 g
Cholesterol ....10 mg
Sodium..........................328 mg
Total Carbohydrate.........33 g
  Dietary Fiber ....9 g
  Sugars ....4 g
Protein ....11 g

Skillet-Roasted Veggie Scramble

After you've tried this dish for dinner, you'll want to have it for breakfast and brunch as well.

Serves 4; 1 stacked tortilla and 1/2 cup cooked vegetables per serving

Vegetable oil spray
1   medium green bell pepper, chopped
1   medium yellow summer squash, diced
1   large onion, chopped
4   ounces sliced button mushrooms
1/2 teaspoon dried oregano, crumbled
1/4 cup water
1/4 teaspoon salt
1/8 teaspoon cayenne
    Egg substitute equivalent to 4 eggs
3   tablespoons fat-free milk
1/4 teaspoon salt
4   6-inch corn tortillas
3/4 cup shredded reduced-fat sharp Cheddar cheese

> **COOK'S TIP**
>
> *If you want to slightly melt the cheese that tops the vegetables, put the tortillas on a broiler rack instead of on plates. Assemble as directed, then run the tortilla stacks under the broiler for about 1 minute.*

1 Heat a 12-inch nonstick skillet over medium-high heat. Remove from the heat and lightly spray with vegetable oil spray (being careful not to spray near a gas flame). Cook the bell pepper, squash, and onion for 3 minutes, stirring occasionally.

2 Stir in the mushrooms and oregano. Cook for 6 minutes, or until just beginning to lightly brown on the edges, stirring constantly. Transfer to a medium bowl.

3 Pour the water into the skillet, scraping the bottom and sides. Stir the water, 1/4 teaspoon salt, and cayenne into the vegetables. Cover to keep warm.

4 In a small bowl, whisk together the egg substitute, milk, and 1/4 teaspoon salt.

5 Lightly spray the skillet with vegetable oil spray. Heat over medium heat. Pour in the egg mixture. Cook without stirring until the mixture begins to set on the bottom and around the edge of the skillet. Using a rubber scraper, lift and fold the partially cooked eggs to allow the uncooked portion to flow underneath. Cook for 1 to 2 minutes, or until the eggs are cooked through but still slightly moist.

6 Place a tortilla on each plate. Spoon the egg mixture onto each tortilla. Top with the vegetables. Sprinkle with the cheese.

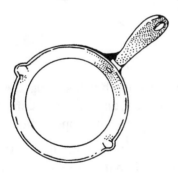

EXCHANGES

1 Starch
1 Lean Meat
2 Vegetable

Calories 180
    Calories from Fat 50
Total Fat...........................6 g
    Saturated Fat ....2.7 g
    Polyunsaturated Fat ....0.6 g
    Monounsaturated Fat .....1.5 g
Cholesterol ....15 mg
Sodium.........................635 mg
Total Carbohydrate........24 g
    Dietary Fiber ....4 g
    Sugars ....7 g
Protein ....15 g

Chunky Vegetable and Egg Salad Sandwiches

Chunky, crunchy vegetables update a classic. Serve it open-face because it's just too much and too good to squeeze between two slices of bread!

Serves 4; heaping 3/4 cup egg salad and 1 slice of toast per serving

- 1/4 cup fat-free or light sour cream
- 2 tablespoons fat-free or light mayonnaise dressing
- 1 tablespoon sweet-pickle relish
- 1/2 tablespoon prepared mustard
- 1/4 teaspoon salt
- 1/8 teaspoon pepper
- 1/8 teaspoon red hot-pepper sauce
- 3 hard-cooked eggs, peeled
- 2 medium ribs of celery, chopped
- 1 medium green bell pepper, chopped
- 4 slices of whole-grain bread (about 1 ounce each), lightly toasted

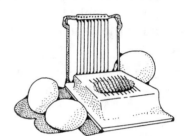

EXCHANGES

1 Starch
1 Very Lean Meat
1 Vegetable

Calories	135
Calories from Fat	23
Total Fat	3 g
Saturated Fat	0.8 g
Polyunsaturated Fat	0.5 g
Monounsaturated Fat	1 g
Cholesterol	54 mg
Sodium	491 mg
Total Carbohydrate	21 g
Dietary Fiber	3 g
Sugars	5 g
Protein	8 g

1 In a medium bowl, stir together the sour cream, mayonnaise, relish, mustard, salt, pepper, and hot-pepper sauce.

2 Cut the eggs in half. Discard two of the yolks. Chop the egg whites and remaining yolks. Add with the celery and bell pepper to the sour cream mixture. Stir to combine.

3 To serve, spoon the egg salad onto the toast.

It's up to you whether to have the toast warm or room temperature. It's the crunch that counts.

COOK'S TIP

Crustless Asparagus and Tomato Quiche

With no crust needed, this quiche is so simple to prepare. Colorful, just slightly sweet grape tomatoes help create a nice balance of flavors and textures.

Serves 6; 1 slice per serving

Vegetable oil spray
1 teaspoon canola oil
6 ounces asparagus, trimmed, sliced on diagonal (about 1 cup)
4 medium green onions (green and white parts), chopped
12 grape tomatoes or cherry tomatoes, halved
Egg substitute equivalent to 2 eggs, or 2 large eggs
1 cup fat-free milk or fat-free evaporated milk
2 teaspoons Dijon mustard
1/2 tablespoon chopped fresh thyme or 1/2 teaspoon dried thyme, crumbled
1/4 teaspoon pepper
1/2 cup shredded or grated reduced-fat Cheddar or Colby cheese

1 Preheat the oven to 350°F. Lightly spray a 9-inch glass pie pan with vegetable oil spray.

2 Heat a medium nonstick skillet over medium heat. Pour in the oil and swirl to coat the bottom. Cook the asparagus and green onions for 4 to 5 minutes, or until soft. Arrange the cooked vegetables and the tomatoes with the cut side down in the pie pan.

3 In a medium bowl, whisk together the remaining ingredients except the cheese. Pour the mixture over the vegetables. Sprinkle with the cheese.

4 Bake for 30 to 35 minutes, or until a knife inserted in the center comes out clean. Let the quiche cool for about 10 minutes before slicing into 6 pieces.

EXCHANGES

1 Very Lean Meat
1/2 Carbohydrate

Calories 61
  Calories from Fat 27
Total Fat.............................3 g
  Saturated Fat ....1.3 g
  Polyunsaturated Fat ....0.3 g
  Monounsaturated Fat .....1.1 g
Cholesterol ....7 mg
Sodium..........................184 mg
Total Carbohydrate...........5 g
  Dietary Fiber ....1 g
  Sugars ....3 g
Protein ....6 g

Italian Eggplant

A slice of eggplant is the base for each serving of this rich-tasting mixture of vegetables, pizza sauce, and creamy cheese.

Serves 4; 1 eggplant stack per serving

    1-pound eggplant, unpeeled
    Vegetable oil spray
1 cup chopped zucchini (about 4 ounces)
1 large onion, chopped
1 medium rib of celery, finely chopped
2 medium garlic cloves, minced
2 teaspoons dried oregano, crumbled
1/4 teaspoon crushed red pepper flakes
1/3 cup water
2 slices whole-wheat bread (about 1 ounce each), processed into very fine crumbs
    Whites of 2 large eggs
1/8 teaspoon salt
1/2 cup pizza sauce
1 cup shredded part-skim mozzarella cheese
2 tablespoons shredded Parmesan cheese

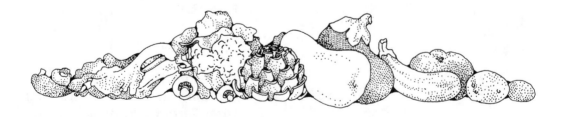

1 Preheat the oven to 350°F.

2 Cut the eggplant crosswise into 1/2-inch slices. Select the 4 largest slices. Lightly spray both sides with vegetable oil spray. Put them on a nonstick baking sheet. Set aside. Chop the remaining eggplant slices into 1/2-inch pieces.

3 Heat a 12-inch nonstick skillet over medium-high heat. Remove from the heat and lightly spray with vegetable oil spray (being careful not to spray near a gas flame). With the skillet still off the heat, stir in the diced eggplant, zucchini, onion, celery, garlic, oregano, and red pepper flakes. Lightly spray with the vegetable oil spray. Cook for 8 minutes, or until the eggplant is tender, stirring frequently. Remove from the heat.

4 Stir in the water, then the bread crumbs, egg whites, and salt. Spoon onto each eggplant slice.

5 Bake for 25 minutes, or until the eggplant rounds are tender. Top each slice with 2 tablespoons pizza sauce. Sprinkle with the mozzarella. Bake for 5 minutes, or until the cheese melts. Remove from the oven.

6 Sprinkle with the Parmesan. Let stand for 5 minutes.

EXCHANGES

1/2 Starch
1 Lean Meat
3 Vegetable
1 Fat

Calories 203
    Calories from Fat 62
Total Fat...........................7 g
    Saturated Fat ....3.8 g
    Polyunsaturated Fat ....0.7 g
    Monounsaturated Fat .....2.0 g
Cholesterol ....18 mg
Sodium...........................580 mg
Total Carbohydrate.........24 g
    Dietary Fiber ....5 g
    Sugars ....11 g
Protein ....14 g

Vegetable Casserole with Dijon-Cheese Sauce

The standing time gives the flavors of the no-bake casserole time to be absorbed and lets the sauce thicken, so don't rush this step. The end result is worth a few minutes' wait.

Serves 6; 1 1/3 cups per serving

1 1/2 pounds red potatoes, thinly sliced
   1 cup fresh or frozen broccoli florets
   1 cup fresh or frozen cauliflower florets
1 1/2 medium carrots, sliced
  1/2 medium red bell pepper, sliced
   2 slices of bread (about 1 ounce each), torn into small pieces

   2 tablespoons cornstarch
1 1/2 cups fat-free milk, divided use
   6 3/4-ounce slices reduced-fat American cheese
   1 teaspoon Dijon mustard
  1/2 teaspoon salt
  1/8 teaspoon cayenne

1 Put a steamer basket in a small amount of simmering water in a Dutch oven. Put the potatoes, broccoli, cauliflower, carrots, and bell pepper in the basket. Cook, covered, for 12 minutes, or until the potatoes are just tender. Transfer to an 11 × 7 × 2-inch baking dish.

2 Meanwhile, preheat the broiler. In a food processor or blender, process the bread until the texture of coarse bread crumbs.

3 In a small bowl, stir together the cornstarch and 1/2 cup milk until the cornstarch is completely dissolved.

4 In a medium saucepan, stir together the remaining 1 cup milk and the cornstarch mixture. Bring to a boil over medium-high heat, stirring frequently with a flat spatula (to scrape the bottom of the pan). Boil until thickened, stirring frequently. Remove from the heat.

5 Stir the cheese, mustard, salt, and cayenne into the sauce until the cheese melts. Pour over the vegetables. Sprinkle with the bread crumbs.

6 Broil for 1 1/2 to 2 minutes, or until browned. Remove from the broiler and let stand for 20 minutes before serving to allow the sauce to thicken slightly.

EXCHANGES

2 Starch	1 Vegetable
1/2 Fat	

Calories 218
Calories from Fat 33
Total Fat .... 4 g
Saturated Fat .... 2.0 g
Polyunsaturated Fat .... 0.4 g
Monounsaturated Fat ..... 1.0 g
Cholesterol .... 11 mg
Sodium .... 590 mg
Total Carbohydrate .... 37 g
Dietary Fiber .... 4 g
Sugars .... 8 g
Protein .... 10 g

Middle Eastern Brown Rice and Pine Nuts

Tender, mildly sweet raisins balance nicely with crunchy pine nuts in this aromatic dish.

Serves 4; 1/2 cup cooked rice and 2/3 cup vegetable mixture per serving

2/3 cup uncooked brown rice
    Vegetable oil spray
1 1/2 large onions, chopped
  1 medium red bell pepper, chopped
  6 ounces vegetable protein (soy) crumbles
1/3 cup pine nuts, dry-roasted
1/4 cup raisins
1/2 teaspoon ground cinnamon
1/4 teaspoon ground allspice, ground nutmeg, or ground cumin
1/4 teaspoon crushed red pepper flakes
1/4 teaspoon salt

1 Prepare the rice using the package directions, omitting the salt and margarine.

2 About 8 minutes before the rice is ready, heat a 12-inch nonstick skillet over medium-high heat. Remove from the heat and lightly spray with vegetable oil spray (being careful not to spray near a gas flame). Put the onions and bell pepper in the skillet. Lightly spray the vegetables with vegetable oil spray. Cook for 6 minutes, or until the vegetables begin to richly brown, stirring frequently.

3 Stir in the remaining ingredients. Cook for 1 minute, or until thoroughly heated.

4 To serve, spoon the rice onto a platter. Spoon the vegetable mixture over the rice.

EXCHANGES

2 Starch
1 Lean Meat
2 Vegetable
1/2 Fruit
1/2 Fat

Calories 318
  Calories from Fat 76
Total Fat...........................8 g
  Saturated Fat ....1.6 g
  Polyunsaturated Fat ....3.4 g
  Monounsaturated Fat .....3.0 g
Cholesterol ....0 mg
Sodium..........................309 mg
Total Carbohydrate.........51 g
  Dietary Fiber ....7 g
  Sugars ....13 g
Protein ....15 g

Lentil Stew with Vegetarian Hot Dogs

A bowl of this satisfying stew, full of vegetables, lentils, and "hot dogs," might very well become a new family favorite.

Serves 4; 1 1/2 cups per serving

- 2 teaspoons olive oil
- 1 cup chopped onion
- 1 cup sliced baby carrots or 2 medium carrots, sliced
- 1 small sweet potato, chopped
- 1 medium rib of celery, sliced
- 1/2 medium green bell pepper, chopped
- 2 medium garlic cloves, minced
- 1/2 cup dried lentils, sorted for stones and shriveled lentils and rinsed
- 1 teaspoon ground cumin
- 1 tablespoon chopped fresh thyme or 1 teaspoon dried thyme, crumbled
- 1/2 teaspoon dry mustard
- 3 cups reduced-sodium vegetable broth or water
- 14.5-ounce can no-salt-added diced tomatoes, undrained
- 2/3 cup water
- 2 bay leaves
- 1/4 teaspoon pepper
- 2 vegetarian hot dogs (about 4 ounces total), sliced, or 4 ounces other vegetarian or meatless sausage, sliced
- 2 tablespoons red wine vinegar

> **COOK'S TIP**
>
> *You can usually find vegetarian hot dogs in the refrigerated section of the supermarket near the fresh produce or in the freezer section. They might also be called soy dogs, soy wieners, veggie dogs, meatless sausage, or vegetarian sausage.*

1 Heat a large saucepan over medium heat. Pour the oil into the saucepan and swirl to coat the bottom. Cook the onion for 3 to 4 minutes, or until tender, stirring frequently.

2 Stir in the carrots, sweet potato, celery, bell pepper, and garlic. Cook for 5 minutes, stirring frequently.

3 Stir in the lentils, cumin, thyme, and mustard. Cook for 1 minute, stirring to coat.

4 Increase the heat to medium high. Stir in the broth, tomatoes, water, bay leaves, and pepper. Bring to a boil. Skim off any foam. Reduce the heat and simmer, covered, for 25 minutes. The lentils will still be firm.

5 Stir in the hot dogs and vinegar. Cook, uncovered, for 5 to 7 minutes, or until the lentils are tender.

6 Remove the bay leaves before serving the stew.

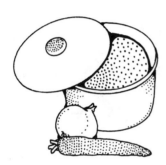

EXCHANGES

1 1/2 Starch
1 Lean Meat
3 Vegetable

Calories	232
Calories from Fat	28
Total Fat	3 g
Saturated Fat	0.4 g
Polyunsaturated Fat	0.5 g
Monounsaturated Fat	1.8 g
Cholesterol	0 mg
Sodium	594 mg
Total Carbohydrate	36 g
Dietary Fiber	11 g
Sugars	11 g
Protein	15 g

Chili-Stuffed Potato Boats

Chili-flavored beans and the usual fixin's top microwaved potatoes.

Serves 4; 1 potato, 2/3 cup vegetable mixture, and 2 tablespoons topping per serving

4 6-ounce baking potatoes (russets preferred)
  Vegetable oil spray
1 medium green bell pepper, chopped
1 large onion, chopped
1/2 15-ounce can no-salt-added pinto beans, rinsed and drained
6 ounces vegetable protein (soy) crumbles
3 tablespoons no-salt-added ketchup
2 teaspoons ground cumin
1/4 teaspoon salt
1/2 cup fat-free or light sour cream
1/2 cup grated reduced-fat sharp Cheddar cheese
1/2 cup finely chopped green onions (green and white parts)

1 Pierce each potato several times with a fork. Microwave the potatoes on 100 percent power (high) for 12 minutes, or until tender when pierced with a fork, turning over once.

2 Meanwhile, heat a large nonstick skillet over medium-high heat. Remove from the heat and lightly spray with vegetable oil spray (being careful not to spray near a gas flame). Cook the bell pepper and onion for 8 minutes, or until beginning to richly brown, stirring occasionally.

3 Stir the beans, vegetable protein crumbles, ketchup, cumin, and salt into the bell pepper mixture. Remove from the heat. Cover and let stand for 5 minutes.

4 To assemble, split the potatoes almost in half lengthwise. Fluff with a fork. Spoon the bean mixture over each potato. Spoon the sour cream, cheese, and green onions over each.

EXCHANGES

3 Starch
1 Very Lean Meat
3 Vegetable

Calories 331
  Calories from Fat 37
Total Fat............................4 g
  Saturated Fat ....1.9 g
  Polyunsaturated Fat ....0.5 g
  Monounsaturated Fat .....1.1 g
Cholesterol ....12 mg
Sodium...........................480 mg
Total Carbohydrate.........60 g
  Dietary Fiber ....10 g
  Sugars ....12 g
Protein ....20 g

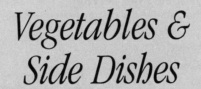

Vegetables & Side Dishes

Pecan-Roasted Asparagus

Roasting brings out the best of both the asparagus and the pecans in this distinctive dish.

Serves 4; about 5 asparagus spears per serving

1 pound asparagus, trimmed
2 tablespoons pecan chips
   Vegetable oil spray
1 tablespoon sugar
1 tablespoon balsamic vinegar
1/4 teaspoon salt

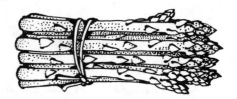

1 Preheat the oven to 425°F.

2 Be sure the asparagus is completely dry. (See Cook's Tip, page 160.) Arrange the asparagus in a single layer on a baking sheet. Sprinkle with the pecans. Lightly spray with the vegetable oil spray.

3 Bake for 10 minutes, or until the asparagus is tender-crisp and the pecans are browned.

4 Meanwhile, in a small bowl, stir together the sugar, vinegar, and salt.

5 Remove the asparagus from the oven. Pour the sugar mixture over the asparagus. Stir gently.

EXCHANGES

1 Vegetable
1/2 Fat

Calories	52
Calories from Fat	25
Total Fat	3 g
Saturated Fat	0.2 g
Polyunsaturated Fat	0.8 g
Monounsaturated Fat	1.5 g
Cholesterol	0 mg
Sodium	151 mg
Total Carbohydrate	6 g
Dietary Fiber	1 g
Sugars	4 g
Protein	2 g

> **COOK'S TIP**
>
> *Be sure to use pecan chips rather than chopped pecans for this recipe. The chips are much smaller and, when roasted, distribute their nutty flavor more evenly over the asparagus. If chips are not available, chop the pecans into very small pieces.*

Asian Broccoli with Pecans

This sweet and nutty side dish is perfect for dressing up a basic entrée of chicken or pork, letting the broccoli get the attention it deserves.

Serves 4; 1/2 cup per serving

2 tablespoons pecan chips
10 ounces fresh or frozen broccoli florets
1 tablespoon sugar
1 tablespoon light soy sauce
1 tablespoon balsamic vinegar
1/2 teaspoon grated peeled gingerroot
1/8 teaspoon crushed red pepper flakes

1 Heat a small skillet over medium-high heat. Dry-roast the pecans for 2 to 3 minutes, or until beginning to lightly brown and become fragrant, stirring frequently. Remove from the heat. Set aside.

2 Set a steamer basket in a small amount of simmering water in a medium saucepan. Put the broccoli in the basket. Cook, covered, for 5 minutes, or until just tender-crisp.

3 Meanwhile, in a small bowl, stir together the remaining ingredients. (It isn't necessary for the sugar to dissolve completely.)

4 To serve, arrange the broccoli on a platter. Spoon the sugar mixture over the broccoli. Sprinkle with the pecans.

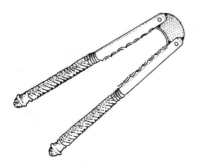

EXCHANGES

1 Vegetable
1/2 Fat

Calories	56
Calories from Fat	25
Total Fat	3 g
Saturated Fat	0.2 g
Polyunsaturated Fat	0.8 g
Monounsaturated Fat	1.6 g
Cholesterol	0 mg
Sodium	156 mg
Total Carbohydrate	7 g
Dietary Fiber	2 g
Sugars	5 g
Protein	2 g

Roasted Green Beans Dijon

These beans are so easy to prepare that you'll want to serve them over and over again.

Serves 6; 1/2 cup per serving

1 pound fresh green beans, trimmed
    Vegetable oil spray
2 teaspoons olive oil
1/2 teaspoon Dijon mustard
1/4 teaspoon salt
1/4 cup snipped fresh parsley

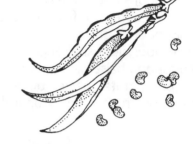

1 Preheat the oven to 425°F.

2 Be sure the beans are thoroughly dry. Put the beans on a nonstick baking sheet. Lightly spray them with vegetable oil spray; toss. Arrange the beans in a single layer on the baking sheet. Spray again.

3 Bake for 10 minutes, or until tender.

4 Meanwhile, in a small bowl, stir together the oil, mustard, and salt.

5 To serve, drizzle the oil mixture over the beans. Stir gently. Sprinkle with the parsley.

EXCHANGES

1 Vegetable

Calories	37
Calories from Fat	16
Total Fat	2 g
Saturated Fat	0.2 g
Polyunsaturated Fat	0.2 g
Monounsaturated Fat	1.1 g
Cholesterol	0 mg
Sodium	110 mg
Total Carbohydrate	5 g
Dietary Fiber	2 g
Sugars	1 g
Protein	1 g

COOK'S TIP

Vegetables that are going to be roasted need to be thoroughly dry. Any moisture will cause them to steam instead of roast and will keep them from browning.

Mediterranean Couscous with Capers

Toss quick-cooking couscous with mild red onions, capers, olive oil, fresh mint, and a splash of lemon. It's so simple, yet so sophisticated.

Serves 7; 1/2 cup per serving

6 ounces uncooked couscous
1/2 cup finely chopped red onion
1/4 cup snipped fresh parsley
1/4 cup finely chopped fresh mint
1/4 cup capers, rinsed and drained
1 1/2 tablespoons olive oil (extra virgin preferred)
1 1/2 tablespoons fresh lemon juice
2 tablespoons fat-free, low-sodium chicken broth
1/2 teaspoon salt
1 medium garlic clove, minced
1/4 teaspoon crushed red pepper flakes
1 teaspoon dried oregano, crumbled (optional)

1 Prepare the couscous using the package directions, omitting the salt and oil. Fluff with a fork.

2 Meanwhile, in a medium bowl, stir together the remaining ingredients.

3 Gently stir the couscous into the onion mixture.

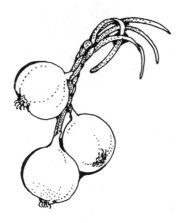

EXCHANGES

1 1/2 Starch
1/2 Fat

Calories	125
Calories from Fat	28
Total Fat	3 g
Saturated Fat	0.4 g
Polyunsaturated Fat	0.3 g
Monounsaturated Fat	2.2 g
Cholesterol	0 mg
Sodium	323 mg
Total Carbohydrate	21 g
Dietary Fiber	2 g
Sugars	2 g
Protein	3 g

Down-Home Greens

Pick your favorite greens—turnip, collard, or mustard—and don't forget the red hot-pepper sauce!

Serves 4; 3/4 cup per serving

14-ounce can low-fat, low-sodium chicken broth
16 ounces frozen chopped turnip, collard, or mustard greens
1 teaspoon dried thyme, crumbled
1/2 teaspoon sugar
1/4 teaspoon crushed red pepper flakes
1/8 teaspoon red hot-pepper sauce, or to taste

1 In a Dutch oven, bring the broth to a boil over high heat.

2 Stir in the remaining ingredients except the hot-pepper sauce. Return to a boil. Reduce the heat and simmer, covered, for 20 minutes, or until tender.

3 Serve with the hot-pepper sauce.

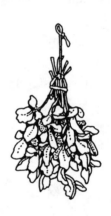

EXCHANGES

1 Vegetable

Calories	43
Calories from Fat	9
Total Fat	1 g
Saturated Fat	0.2 g
Polyunsaturated Fat	0.3 g
Monounsaturated Fat	0.2 g
Cholesterol	2 mg
Sodium	60 mg
Total Carbohydrate	6 g
Dietary Fiber	4 g
Sugars	1 g
Protein	4 g

Mushrooms Marinated in Lime and Soy Sauce

A perfect accompaniment for grilled steaks or chicken, these mushrooms are also delicious served uncooked as an appetizer. Just drain, toss with parsley, and serve.

Serves 8; 4 mushrooms per serving

    1 pound whole button mushrooms (about 32)
 1/4 cup light soy sauce
 1/4 cup fresh lime juice
    1 tablespoon olive oil
 1/4 teaspoon crushed red pepper flakes
        Vegetable oil spray
    2 medium limes, quartered
 1/4 cup snipped fresh parsley

1   In a large airtight plastic bag, stir together the mushrooms, soy sauce, lime juice, oil, and red pepper flakes. Seal the bag and turn to coat the mushrooms evenly. Refrigerate for about 8 hours, turning occasionally.

2   For a side dish, preheat the broiler. Lightly spray a nonstick baking sheet with vegetable oil spray. Drain the mushrooms, discarding the marinade. Arrange the mushrooms in a single layer on the baking sheet.

3   Broil the mushrooms 4 to 6 inches from the heat for 6 minutes, or until beginning to brown, stirring occasionally.

4   For an appetizer, drain the mushrooms, discarding the marinade.

5   For both the broiled and the raw mushrooms, squeeze the lime over the mushrooms. Sprinkle with the parsley.

EXCHANGES

1 Vegetable

Calories 21
  Calories from Fat 6
Total Fat .... 1 g
  Saturated Fat .... 0.1 g
  Polyunsaturated Fat .... 0.1 g
  Monounsaturated Fat ..... 0.3 g
Cholesterol .... 0 mg
Sodium .... 75 mg
Total Carbohydrate .... 3 g
  Dietary Fiber .... 1 g
  Sugars .... 1 g
Protein .... 1 g

Lemon-Mint Sugar Snaps

Delicate sugar snaps coupled with fresh lemon and mint are definitely a true taste of spring.

Serves 5; 1/2 cup per serving

- 8 ounces sugar snap peas, trimmed
- 1/2 teaspoon grated lemon zest
- 2 tablespoons fresh lemon juice
- 1 tablespoon light tub margarine
- 1/8 teaspoon salt
- 1/4 cup chopped fresh mint or snipped fresh cilantro

1 Set a steamer basket in a small amount of simmering water in a medium saucepan. Put the peas in the basket. Cook, covered, for 5 minutes, or until just tender-crisp. Pour into a medium bowl.

2 Meanwhile, in a small bowl, stir together the remaining ingredients except the mint.

3 Gently stir the lemon mixture and mint into the peas.

EXCHANGES

1 Vegetable

Calories	30
Calories from Fat	9
Total Fat	1 g
Saturated Fat	0.0 g
Polyunsaturated Fat	0.2 g
Monounsaturated Fat	0.5 g
Cholesterol	0 mg
Sodium	81 mg
Total Carbohydrate	4 g
Dietary Fiber	1 g
Sugars	2 g
Protein	1 g

Red Potatoes Parmesan

These moist, tender potatoes are tossed with a mixture of Parmesan, margarine, fresh parsley, and green onions.

Serves 4; 1/2 cup per serving

12 ounces red potatoes, cut into 1/2-inch cubes
2 tablespoons light tub margarine
2 tablespoons snipped fresh parsley
1/4 cup minced green onions (green and white parts)
1/4 teaspoon salt
2 tablespoons shredded Parmesan cheese

1 Set a steamer basket in a small amount of simmering water in a saucepan. Put the potatoes in the basket. Cook, covered, for 8 minutes, or until tender when pierced with a fork. Drain.

2 In a medium bowl, gently stir together the cooked potatoes and the remaining ingredients except the Parmesan.

3 Gently stir in the Parmesan.

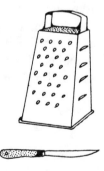

EXCHANGES

1 Starch
1/2 Fat

Calories 106
  Calories from Fat 29
Total Fat..............................3 g
  Saturated Fat ....0.5 g
  Polyunsaturated Fat ....0.6 g
  Monounsaturated Fat .....1.6 g
Cholesterol ....3 mg
Sodium..........................218 mg
Total Carbohydrate.........17 g
  Dietary Fiber ....2 g
  Sugars ....2 g
Protein ....3 g

Scalloped Potatoes

Just slice, layer, and bake—how can something so easy taste so good?

Serves 6; 1/2 cup per serving

Vegetable oil spray
1 pound russet potatoes, thinly sliced
1/4 cup finely chopped onion
2 tablespoons light tub margarine
1/4 teaspoon salt
1/8 teaspoon pepper
1/4 cup grated part-skim mozzarella cheese or reduced-fat sharp Cheddar cheese
1/2 cup fat-free milk, warmed
1/4 teaspoon salt
1/4 cup grated part-skim mozzarella cheese or reduced-fat sharp Cheddar cheese

1 Preheat the oven to 425°F.

2 Lightly spray a 9-inch glass pie pan with vegetable oil spray. Arrange half the potato slices in the pie pan. Top with the onion, dots of margarine, 1/4 teaspoon salt, pepper, and 1/4 cup cheese. Top with the remaining potatoes. Pour the milk over all.

3 Bake, uncovered, for 30 minutes. Sprinkle with the remaining 1/4 teaspoon salt and the remaining 1/4 cup cheese. Bake for 5 minutes, or until the cheese has melted. Remove from the oven. Let stand for 5 minutes.

EXCHANGES

1 Starch
1/2 Fat

Calories	108
Calories from Fat	27
Total Fat	3 g
Saturated Fat	1.0 g
Polyunsaturated Fat	0.4 g
Monounsaturated Fat	1.3 g
Cholesterol	6 mg
Sodium	284 mg
Total Carbohydrate	16 g
Dietary Fiber	2 g
Sugars	3 g
Protein	5 g

Russet potatoes will absorb the moisture in this dish, providing the desired starchiness.

Brown-Sugar-and-Spice Sweet Potatoes

A combination of dark brown sugar, spices, and margarine melts over sweet potatoes for a delightfully aromatic side dish.

Serves 4; 1/2 sweet potato and 1/2 tablespoon margarine mixture per serving

2 8-ounce sweet potatoes
1 1/2 tablespoons light tub margarine
1 tablespoon firmly packed dark brown sugar
1/2 teaspoon grated orange zest
1/4 teaspoon ground cinnamon
1/4 teaspoon vanilla extract
1/8 teaspoon salt
Dash of ground allspice, nutmeg, or cloves

1 Pierce the potatoes in several places with a fork. Microwave on 100 percent power (high) for 8 minutes, or until tender when pierced with a fork. Cut in half lengthwise. Fluff with a fork.

2 Meanwhile, in a small bowl, stir together the remaining ingredients.

3 To serve, spoon the margarine mixture over the potatoes.

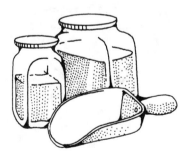

EXCHANGES

1 1/2 Starch

Calories 103
Calories from Fat 16
Total Fat............................2 g
Saturated Fat ....0.0 g
Polyunsaturated Fat ....0.4 g
Monounsaturated Fat .....0.9 g
Cholesterol ....0 mg
Sodium..........................112 mg
Total Carbohydrate........21 g
Dietary Fiber ....2 g
Sugars ....12 g
Protein ....1 g

Red Pepper Pilaf

Red bell peppers, turmeric, and parsley color this dish, which has a risottolike texture.

Serves 6; 1/2 cup per serving

1 1/4 cups water
2/3 cup uncooked brown rice
2 medium red bell peppers, cut into 1-inch pieces
1 cup chopped onion
1/2 teaspoon ground turmeric
1/4 teaspoon crushed red pepper flakes
1/2 cup snipped fresh parsley
1 tablespoon olive oil
1/2 teaspoon salt

1 In a medium saucepan, bring the water to a boil over high heat. Stir in the rice, bell peppers, onion, turmeric, and red pepper flakes. Return to a boil. Reduce the heat and simmer, covered, for 40 minutes, or until the rice is tender and the liquid is absorbed. Remove from the heat.

2 Stir in the remaining ingredients.

EXCHANGES

1 Starch
1 Vegetable
1/2 Fat

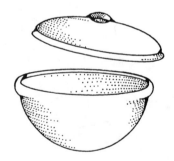

Calories 122
Calories from Fat 27
Total Fat...........................3 g
Saturated Fat ....0.4 g
Polyunsaturated Fat ....0.5 g
Monounsaturated Fat .....1.9 g
Cholesterol ....0 mg
Sodium...........................200 mg
Total Carbohydrate.........22 g
Dietary Fiber ....2 g
Sugars ....3 g
Protein ....3 g

Toasted-Almond Rice and Peas

Rice tossed with green peas and crunchy almonds is a perfect side for Asian fare or a simple roast chicken.

Serves 6; 1/2 cup per serving

1 1/3 cups water
2/3 cup uncooked brown rice
1/2 teaspoon ground turmeric
3 tablespoons sliced almonds
3/4 cup frozen green peas, thawed
1/4 cup finely chopped green onions
   (green and white parts)
1/2 teaspoon salt

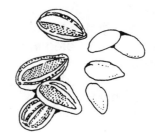

1 In a medium saucepan, bring the water to a boil over high heat. Stir in the rice and turmeric. Return to a boil. Reduce the heat and simmer, covered, for 30 minutes, or until the rice is tender and the liquid is absorbed.

2 Meanwhile, heat a medium skillet over medium-high heat. Dry-roast the almonds for 2 to 3 minutes, stirring constantly. Remove from the heat.

3 When the rice is cooked, stir in the remaining ingredients, including the almonds.

COOK'S TIP

Save some time by dry-roasting the nuts for several recipes at once. Let them cool completely, then store them in an airtight container at room temperature for up to two weeks.

EXCHANGES

1 1/2 Starch

Calories 120
  Calories from Fat 27
Total Fat..............................3 g
  Saturated Fat ....0.3 g
  Polyunsaturated Fat ....0.8 g
  Monounsaturated Fat .....1.7 g
Cholesterol ....0 mg
Sodium........................213 mg
Total Carbohydrate........20 g
  Dietary Fiber ....2 g
  Sugars ....2 g
Protein ....4 g

Italian Skillet Spinach

From the time this hits the skillet to the time it hits the serving bowl is about *one minute*. Speed cooking at its best!

Serves 4; 1/2 cup per serving

2 tablespoons light tub margarine
1 teaspoon grated lemon zest
1 teaspoon dried oregano, crumbled
1/4 teaspoon salt
1/8 teaspoon crushed red pepper flakes
9 ounces spinach
3 tablespoons water

1 In a small bowl, stir together the margarine, lemon zest, oregano, salt, and red pepper flakes.

2 Heat a 12-inch nonstick skillet over medium-high heat. Put the spinach and water in the skillet. Cook for 1 minute, or until tender, tossing constantly with two utensils. Remove from the heat.

3 Stir in the margarine mixture.

EXCHANGES

1 Vegetable
1/2 Fat

Calories	36
Calories from Fat	22
Total Fat	2 g
Saturated Fat	0.0 g
Polyunsaturated Fat	0.6 g
Monounsaturated Fat	1.3 g
Cholesterol	0 mg
Sodium	242 mg
Total Carbohydrate	2 g
Dietary Fiber	2 g
Sugars	0 g
Protein	2 g

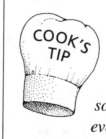

COOK'S TIP

Fresh spinach cooks down rapidly. Toss or stir it constantly so it will cook evenly.

Acorn Squash Filled with Dried Apricots and Plums

With their filling of dried fruit and spices, these acorn squash provide the perfect festive touch to a holiday table, dinner party, or Sunday dinner.

Serves 4; 1/2 squash per serving

Vegetable oil spray
2 acorn squash (about 1 pound each), halved and seeded
1/2 cup dried apricots, chopped
1/4 cup orange-flavor dried plums, chopped
1/4 cup fresh orange juice
1 teaspoon ground cinnamon
1/4 teaspoon ground allspice or ground nutmeg
2 tablespoons light tub margarine

1 Preheat the oven to 350°F. Lightly spray a 13 × 9 × 2-inch baking pan with vegetable oil spray.

2 Pierce the skin of the squash in several places with a fork or the tip of a sharp knife. Put the squash with the cut side up in the baking pan.

3 In a small bowl, stir together the remaining ingredients except the margarine. Spoon into the squash cavities. Cover the pan with aluminum foil.

4 Bake for 1 hour 15 minutes, or until the squash is tender when the flesh is pierced with a fork. Remove from the oven.

5 Dot the margarine over the filling in each squash half. Let the margarine melt before serving the squash.

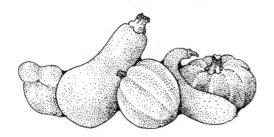

EXCHANGES

1 1/2 Starch
1 Fruit

Calories 162
Calories from Fat 23
Total Fat..............................3 g
Saturated Fat ....0.0 g
Polyunsaturated Fat ....0.6 g
Monounsaturated Fat .....1.3 g
Cholesterol ....0 mg
Sodium...........................53 mg
Total Carbohydrate.........36 g
Dietary Fiber ....8 g
Sugars ....18 g
Protein ....2 g

Thyme-Tinged Squash

A bit of sugar brings out the naturally sweet taste of the squash and onion and also helps the vegetables brown lightly.

Serves 6; 1/2 cup per serving

    Vegetable oil spray
1 pound yellow summer squash, sliced
1 large onion, chopped
1 teaspoon sugar
1/2 teaspoon dried thyme, crumbled
2 tablespoons light tub margarine
1/2 teaspoon salt

1 Heat a large nonstick skillet over medium-high heat. Remove from the heat and lightly spray with vegetable oil spray (being careful not to spray near a gas flame). Put the squash, onion, sugar, and thyme in the skillet. Lightly spray the vegetables with vegetable oil spray. Cook for 8 minutes, or until the squash is tender and beginning to richly brown, stirring frequently. Remove from the heat.

2 Stir in the margarine and salt.

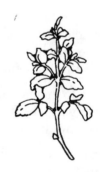

EXCHANGES

1 Vegetable
1/2 Fat

Calories	45
Calories from Fat	15
Total Fat	2 g
Saturated Fat	0.0 g
Polyunsaturated Fat	0.4 g
Monounsaturated Fat	0.9 g
Cholesterol	0 mg
Sodium	226 mg
Total Carbohydrate	7 g
Dietary Fiber	2 g
Sugars	5 g
Protein	1 g

Zucchini Sticks

Instead of masking its flavor by frying zucchini and then dipping it in a heavy sauce, try this recipe for baked zucchini sticks. It lets the fresh taste shine.

Serves 4; 2 pieces per serving

1/3 cup fat-free Italian salad dressing
1/2 cup yellow cornmeal
1/2 teaspoon paprika
    Vegetable oil spray
  2 medium zucchini, quartered lengthwise
1/4 teaspoon salt
  1 medium lemon, cut into eighths

1 Preheat the oven to 425°F.

2 Pour the salad dressing into a shallow bowl or pie pan.

3 In another shallow dish or pie pan, stir together the cornmeal and paprika. Place the containers side by side.

4 Lightly spray a nonstick cookie sheet with vegetable oil spray. Place the cookie sheet beside the cornmeal mixture.

5 Roll a piece of zucchini in the salad dressing to coat completely. Let the excess drip off. Roll in the cornmeal. Shake off the excess. Place on the cookie sheet. Repeat with the remaining zucchini. Lightly spray with vegetable oil spray.

6 Bake for 10 minutes. Gently turn over and bake for 2 minutes. Turn again and bake for 2 more minutes, or until golden and just tender. Remove from the oven. Sprinkle with the salt.

7 To serve, place the zucchini sticks on plates. Serve with the lemon wedges to squeeze over the zucchini.

EXCHANGES

1/2 Starch
1 Vegetable

Calories	70
Calories from Fat	4
Total Fat	0 g
Saturated Fat	0.0 g
Polyunsaturated Fat	0.2 g
Monounsaturated Fat	0.1 g
Cholesterol	0 mg
Sodium	303 mg
Total Carbohydrate	15 g
Dietary Fiber	2 g
Sugars	3 g
Protein	2 g

Mediterranean Zucchini

To put a touch of sophistication on your menu without much effort, serve this dish at your next dinner party. Be prepared for lots of ooohs and ahhhs.

Serves 4; 1/2 zucchini per serving

2 medium zucchini (5 to 6 ounces each), trimmed and cut in half lengthwise
2 teaspoons olive oil
1/2 teaspoon grated lemon zest
1/2 teaspoon dried basil, crumbled
1/2 teaspoon dried oregano, crumbled
1/8 teaspoon crushed red pepper flakes
1/8 teaspoon salt
1 tablespoon plus 1 teaspoon shredded Parmesan cheese

1 Preheat the oven to 400°F.

2 Place the zucchini with the cut side up on a baking sheet. Drizzle 1/2 teaspoon of the oil over each half.

3 In a small bowl, stir together the remaining ingredients except the Parmesan. Sprinkle over the zucchini.

4 Bake for 20 minutes, or just until tender. Remove from the oven.

5 Sprinkle with the Parmesan. Let stand for 5 minutes before serving.

EXCHANGES

1 Vegetable
1/2 Fat

Calories 43
Calories from Fat 27
Total Fat..............................3 g
Saturated Fat ....0.6 g
Polyunsaturated Fat ....0.3 g
Monounsaturated Fat .....1.9 g
Cholesterol ....2 mg
Sodium................................87 mg
Total Carbohydrate...........3 g
Dietary Fiber ....1 g
Sugars ....2 g
Protein ....2 g

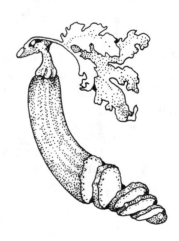

Tarragon Tomatoes

By using this combination of ingredients to raise the flavor a notch, you can enjoy tomatoes even in the off-season.

Serves 4; 1 tomato per serving

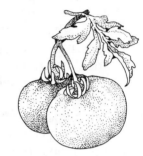

2 tablespoons fat-free or light mayonnaise dressing
1/2 tablespoon Dijon mustard
1 teaspoon prepared white horseradish
1/2 teaspoon dried tarragon, crumbled
4 medium tomatoes
1/2 cup soft bread crumbs (whole wheat preferred)
Vegetable oil spray (olive oil spray preferred)

1 Preheat the oven to 350°F.

2 In a small bowl, stir together the mayonnaise, mustard, horseradish, and tarragon.

3 Cut a 1/4-inch slice from the stem end and a very thin slice from the bottom of each tomato. Place the tomatoes with the stem end up in a pie pan.

4 To assemble, spread the mayonnaise mixture over each tomato. Top each with 2 tablespoons bread crumbs. Lightly spray the bread crumbs with vegetable oil spray.

5 Bake for 30 minutes, or until the tomatoes are just tender in the center when pierced with a fork. Remove from the oven. Let stand for 5 minutes before serving.

COOK'S TIP

Cutting the thin slice off the bottom of each tomato keeps the tomatoes from tilting. Be careful not to slice too deep, or you'll allow the juices to escape.

EXCHANGES

2 Vegetable

Calories 58
Calories from Fat 7
Total Fat..............................1 g
Saturated Fat ....0.0 g
Polyunsaturated Fat ....0.2 g
Monounsaturated Fat .....0.2 g
Cholesterol ....0 mg
Sodium..........................152 mg
Total Carbohydrate.........12 g
Dietary Fiber ....2 g
Sugars ....5 g
Protein ....2 g

Veggie Stir-Fry, Mexican Style

This colorful stir-fry is great with broiled or skillet-grilled chicken or pork.

Serves 5; 1/2 cup per serving

Vegetable oil spray
1 poblano pepper or 1 medium green bell pepper, seeds and ribs discarded, cut in thin strips
1/2 cup matchstick-size carrot strips
1/2 medium onion, thinly sliced
1 1/2 cups frozen whole-kernel corn, thawed, drained, and patted dry with paper towels
1 1/2 tablespoons light tub margarine
1/2 teaspoon chili powder
1/2 teaspoon ground cumin
1/4 teaspoon dried oregano, crumbled
1/4 teaspoon salt
1/8 teaspoon crushed red pepper flakes

1 Heat a 12-inch nonstick skillet over medium-high heat. Remove from the heat and lightly spray with vegetable oil spray (being careful not to spray near a gas flame). Cook the poblano, carrots, and onion for 7 to 8 minutes, or until beginning to brown on the edges, stirring frequently.

2 Stir in the corn. Cook for 1 minute, stirring frequently. Remove the skillet from the heat.

3 Stir in the remaining ingredients.

EXCHANGES

1/2 Starch
1 Vegetable

Calories 70
  Calories from Fat 16
Total Fat.............................2 g
  Saturated Fat ....0.0 g
  Polyunsaturated Fat ....0.5 g
  Monounsaturated Fat .....0.9 g
Cholesterol ....0 mg
Sodium................................155 mg
Total Carbohydrate.........14 g
  Dietary Fiber ....2 g
  Sugars ....3 g
Protein ....2 g

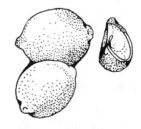

Nutmeg-Spiced Vegetable Medley

Nutmeg and cumin blend to provide a mildly spiced seasoning for a trio of steamed vegetables.

Serves 4; 2/3 cup per serving

1 cup sliced carrots
1 cup cauliflower florets
1 cup broccoli florets
2 tablespoons light tub margarine
1 teaspoon sugar
1/4 teaspoon ground cumin
1/4 teaspoon salt
1/8 teaspoon ground nutmeg
Dash of cayenne

1 Set a steamer basket in a small amount of simmering water in a medium saucepan. Put the carrots, cauliflower, and broccoli in the basket. Cook, covered, for 5 minutes, or until just tender-crisp. Put in a medium bowl.

2 Meanwhile, in a small bowl, stir together the remaining ingredients.

3 Stir the margarine mixture into the cooked vegetables.

EXCHANGES

1 Vegetable
1/2 Fat

Calories 49
  Calories from Fat 22
Total Fat.............................2 g
  Saturated Fat ....0.0 g
  Polyunsaturated Fat ....0.6 g
  Monounsaturated Fat .....1.3 g
Cholesterol ....0 mg
Sodium...........................214 mg
Total Carbohydrate...........6 g
  Dietary Fiber ....2 g
  Sugars ....4 g
Protein ....1 g

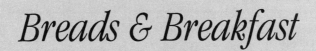

Breads & Breakfast

Rosemary and Dill Quick Bread

Even the novice cook can prepare this bread with confidence. It goes together quickly and requires no rising time.

Serves 16; 1 slice per serving

Vegetable oil spray
2 cups all-purpose flour
1 cup whole-wheat flour
1 teaspoon dried dill weed, crumbled
1 teaspoon dried rosemary, crushed
1 teaspoon baking soda
1/2 teaspoon baking powder
1/2 teaspoon garlic powder
1/2 teaspoon salt
1 1/3 cups fat-free or low-fat buttermilk
3 tablespoons honey
2 tablespoons olive oil

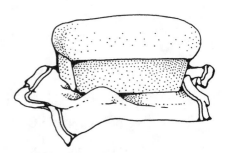

1 Preheat the oven to 350°F. Lightly spray a baking sheet with vegetable oil spray.

2 In a large bowl, stir together both flours, dill weed, rosemary, baking soda, baking powder, garlic powder, and salt.

3 Add the remaining ingredients. Stir only until moistened.

4 Shape the dough into a ball. Put the dough on a flat surface and knead gently for about 5 seconds. Put the dough on the baking sheet. Shape the dough into an oval loaf, about 8 × 6 inches. Slightly flatten the top. With a sharp knife, cut 4 diagonal slashes about 1/4 inch deep across the top of the bread. This will prevent cracking during baking.

5 Bake, uncovered, for 40 to 45 minutes, or until the loaf is golden brown, sounds hollow when tapped, and registers 190°F on an instant-read thermometer.

6 Remove from the pan and let cool for 10 to 15 minutes on a cooling rack before slicing.

EXCHANGES

1 1/2 Starch

Calories	110
Calories from Fat	11
Total Fat	1 g
Saturated Fat	0.2 g
Polyunsaturated Fat	0.2 g
Monounsaturated Fat	0.7 g
Cholesterol	0 mg
Sodium	174 mg
Total Carbohydrate	22 g
Dietary Fiber	1 g
Sugars	5 g
Protein	3 g

Lemon-Lime Poppy Seed Muffins

Moist and satisfying with the delicate crunch of poppy seeds, these muffins are a sure-fire way to start your morning on the right track.

Serves 12; 1 muffin per serving

Vegetable oil spray
2 cups all-purpose flour
1/2 cup firmly packed light brown sugar
1 tablespoon poppy seeds
2 teaspoons baking powder
1/2 teaspoon baking soda
1/4 teaspoon salt
Egg substitute equivalent to 1 egg, or 1 large egg
3/4 cup fat-free milk
2 tablespoons honey
1 tablespoon canola oil
2 teaspoons grated lemon zest
1 tablespoon fresh lemon juice
2 teaspoons grated lime zest

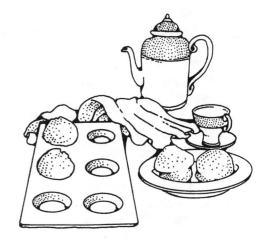

1 Preheat the oven to 375°F. Lightly spray a 12-cup muffin tin with vegetable oil spray.

2 In a large bowl, stir together the flour, brown sugar, poppy seeds, baking powder, baking soda, and salt. Make a well in the center of the mixture.

3 Put the remaining ingredients in the well. Stir just until moistened. Don't overmix; the batter will be slightly lumpy. Put about 1/4 cup batter in each muffin cup.

4 Bake for 15 to 17 minutes, or until a toothpick inserted in the center comes out clean. Put the muffin tin on a cooling rack and let cool for about 10 minutes before serving the muffins.

EXCHANGES

2 Carbohydrate

Calories	144
Calories from Fat	15
Total Fat	2 g
Saturated Fat	0.2 g
Polyunsaturated Fat	0.6 g
Monounsaturated Fat	0.7 g
Cholesterol	0 mg
Sodium	182 mg
Total Carbohydrate	29 g
Dietary Fiber	1 g
Sugars	13 g
Protein	3 g

Apple Crumble Coffee Cake

Coffee cake with a crisp crumbled topping and a surprise of tender apples on the bottom—what a lovely way to begin your day! (See photo insert.)

Serves 16; 1 square per serving

Vegetable oil spray
2 medium Granny Smith apples, peeled and thinly sliced
2 tablespoons unsweetened apple juice
1 tablespoon honey
1 teaspoon ground cinnamon
1 1/2 cups all-purpose flour
1/3 cup sugar
2 1/2 teaspoons baking powder
1/2 cup fat-free milk
1/4 cup unsweetened applesauce
Egg substitute equivalent
to 1 egg, or 1 large egg
1 tablespoon canola oil
1/2 cup uncooked quick-cooking oatmeal
3 tablespoons light brown sugar
3 tablespoons chopped pecans
1 teaspoon ground cinnamon
2 tablespoons light tub margarine, softened

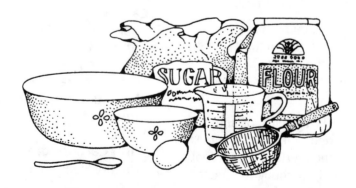

1 Preheat the oven to 375°F. Lightly spray an 8-inch square baking pan with vegetable oil spray. Set aside.

2 Heat a medium nonstick skillet over medium heat. Cook the apples and apple juice for 4 to 5 minutes, or until the apples are tender-crisp, stirring occasionally.

3 Stir in the honey and cinnamon. Cook for 1 to 2 minutes, or until the cinnamon is distributed throughout the apples and the mixture is warmed through, stirring occasionally.

4 Put the prepared pan on a cooling rack. Pour the apple mixture into the pan. Let cool for 5 minutes.

5 In a medium bowl, stir together the flour, sugar, and baking powder. Make a well in the center.

6 Add the milk, applesauce, egg substitute, and canola oil to the well, stirring just until the flour mixture is moistened. Don't overmix; the batter will be slightly lumpy.

7 In a small bowl, stir together the remaining ingredients with a fork. Sprinkle over the coffee cake.

8 Bake for 25 to 30 minutes, or until a toothpick inserted in the center comes out clean. Let the pan cool on a cooling rack for 15 minutes before cutting the coffee cake into squares.

EXCHANGES

1/2 Fat
1 1/2 Carbohydrate

Calories	120
Calories from Fat	25
Total Fat	3 g
Saturated Fat	0.2 g
Polyunsaturated Fat	0.8 g
Monounsaturated Fat	1.5 g
Cholesterol	0 mg
Sodium	81 mg
Total Carbohydrate	22 g
Dietary Fiber	1 g
Sugars	11 g
Protein	2 g

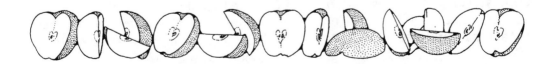

Apricot and Apple Granola

Making your own homemade granola is fun. Let the family help measure, mix, and bake. Then pack the cooled mixture into small airtight bags for a quick breakfast or snack on the go.

Serves 16; 1/2 cup per serving

Vegetable oil spray
4 cups uncooked quick-cooking oatmeal
1/2 cup toasted wheat germ
1/2 cup firmly packed light brown sugar
1 teaspoon ground cinnamon
1/2 cup water
1/2 cup apricot nectar
2 tablespoons honey
1 tablespoon canola oil
2 cups bran cereal (buds or flakes)
1/2 cup chopped dried apricots
1/2 cup chopped dried apples

COOK'S TIP

While the granola is still warm, try some with fat-free milk poured on top. Then store what's left in an airtight container or plastic bags at room temperature for up to two weeks.

1 Preheat the oven to 300°F. Lightly spray a rimmed baking sheet with vegetable oil spray.

EXCHANGES

2 1/2 Carbohydrate

Calories	179
Calories from Fat	24
Total Fat	3 g
Saturated Fat	0.4 g
Polyunsaturated Fat	1.0 g
Monounsaturated Fat	1.0 g
Cholesterol	0 mg
Sodium	71 mg
Total Carbohydrate	37 g
Dietary Fiber	6 g
Sugars	16 g
Protein	5 g

2 In a large bowl, stir together the oatmeal, wheat germ, brown sugar, almonds, and cinnamon.

3 In a small bowl, whisk together the water, apricot nectar, honey, and vegetable oil. Pour into the oatmeal mixture. Stir until all the oatmeal mixture is moistened. Spread on the baking sheet.

4 Bake for 1 hour, or until the mixture is toasted and lightly golden brown, stirring every 20 minutes. Put the baking sheet on a cooling rack. Let the mixture cool for 30 minutes.

5 Stir in the bran cereal, apricots, and apples.

Apple Pie Breakfast Parfaits

Apple pie for breakfast? When cinnamon-scented apple slices are layered with vanilla yogurt, then topped with golden raisins and toasted walnuts, this crustless version fits the bill.

Serves 6; 1 cup per serving

    20-ounce can unsweetened sliced apples, drained
1 tablespoon honey
1/2 teaspoon ground cinnamon
1 teaspoon grated lemon zest
1 teaspoon fresh lemon juice
4 cups fat-free or low-fat vanilla yogurt
4 tablespoons golden raisins
3 tablespoons chopped walnuts, dry-roasted

1 In a small bowl, stir together the drained apples, honey, cinnamon, lemon zest, and lemon juice.

2 To assemble, spoon about 2 1/2 tablespoons apple mixture into each parfait glass or other clear glass. Spoon 1/3 cup yogurt on the apple mixture in each glass. Repeat the layers. Sprinkle each serving with raisins and walnuts.

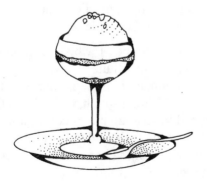

EXCHANGES

1 Fruit
1 Fat-Free Milk
1/2 Fat

Calories	168
Calories from Fat	20
Total Fat	2 g
Saturated Fat	0.2 g
Polyunsaturated Fat	1.2 g
Monounsaturated Fat	0.5 g
Cholesterol	3 mg
Sodium	95 mg
Total Carbohydrate	31 g
Dietary Fiber	2 g
Sugars	24 g
Protein	7 g

French Toast Casserole with Honey-Glazed Fruit

Make weekend time special time with this lightly sweetened French toast casserole.

Serves 4; 1 cup per serving

Vegetable oil spray
6 slices whole-wheat bread
(about 1 ounce each), cut in half
vertically
1 1/2 cups fat-free milk
Egg substitute equivalent to 6 eggs
2 tablespoons light brown sugar
1 teaspoon ground cinnamon
1/4 teaspoon ground nutmeg
15-ounce can light fruit cocktail,
drained
2 tablespoons honey
1 tablespoon light tub margarine

COOK'S TIP

If you prepare this casserole ahead of time, cover it with plastic wrap and refrigerate for up to 10 hours. Put the cold casserole in a cold oven, set the thermostat to 350°F, and bake for 65 to 70 minutes, or until the center is set.

1 Preheat the oven to 350°F. Lightly spray an 8-inch square baking pan with vegetable oil spray.

EXCHANGES

1 Very Lean Meat
3 1/2 Carbohydrate

Calories	286
Calories from Fat	27
Total Fat	3 g
Saturated Fat	0.5 g
Polyunsaturated Fat	0.7 g
Monounsaturated Fat	1.4 g
Cholesterol	2 mg
Sodium	469 mg
Total Carbohydrate	49 g
Dietary Fiber	4 g
Sugars	30 g
Protein	16 g

2 Place the bread with the cut sides (the crustless side) touching the bottom of the pan and the crust sides overlapping each other slightly. The slices should be almost flat. Set aside.

3 In a medium bowl, whisk together the milk, egg substitute, brown sugar, cinnamon, and nutmeg. Pour over the bread. Using a spoon, press down the bread to soak up the milk mixture. Spread the fruit cocktail over the bread. Drizzle with the honey. Dot with the margarine.

4 Bake, uncovered, for 55 to 60 minutes, or until the center is set (doesn't jiggle when gently shaken). Let cool for at least 10 minutes before cutting.

Ham-and-Swiss Breakfast Casserole

Perfect for a brunch, this casserole combines the texture of a classic egg casserole and the flavors of ham and Swiss on rye.

Serves 6; 3/4 cup per serving

Vegetable oil spray
4 slices rye bread (about 1 ounce each), cut into 1/2-inch cubes (about 3 cups cubes)
3 ounces lower-sodium, low-fat ham, diced (about 1/2 cup)
1/2 medium red bell pepper, diced
2 ounces reduced-fat Swiss cheese, diced (about 1/4 cup)
2 cups fat-free milk
Egg substitute equivalent to 4 eggs
2 tablespoons shredded Parmesan cheese
1/2 teaspoon dry mustard
1/2 teaspoon onion powder
1/4 teaspoon black pepper

If you prepare this casserole ahead of time, cover it with plastic wrap and refrigerate for up to 10 hours. Put the cold casserole in a cold oven, set the thermostat to 350°F, and bake for 65 to 70 minutes, or until the center is set.

1 Preheat the oven to 350°F. Lightly spray an 8-inch square baking pan with vegetable oil spray.

2 Put the bread cubes, ham, bell pepper, and Swiss cheese in the pan, stirring 3 or 4 times to combine.

3 In a medium bowl, whisk together the remaining ingredients. Pour over the bread mixture, pressing the bread down with a spoon to soak up the milk mixture.

4 Bake, uncovered, for 55 to 60 minutes, or until the center is set (doesn't jiggle when gently shaken). Let cool for at least 10 minutes before cutting into 6 pieces.

EXCHANGES

1/2 Starch
1 Lean Meat
1/2 Fat-Free Milk

Calories 149
  Calories from Fat 25
Total Fat.............................3 g
  Saturated Fat ....1.3 g
  Polyunsaturated Fat ....0.3 g
  Monounsaturated Fat .....0.9 g
Cholesterol ....13 mg
Sodium...........................411 mg
Total Carbohydrate.........15 g
  Dietary Fiber ....1 g
  Sugars ....6 g
Protein ....15 g

Southwestern Breakfast Tortilla Wrap

Make a batch of these wraps ahead of time so you can zap one in the microwave for a fast, filling breakfast.

Serves 6; 1 tortilla and 1/2 cup filling per serving

   4 ounces low-fat turkey breakfast sausage links, casings removed
   6 6-inch low-fat whole-wheat tortillas
     Vegetable oil spray
   2 cups frozen whole-kernel corn
     Egg substitute equivalent
     to 4 eggs, or 4 large eggs
1/4 teaspoon chili powder
1/4 cup salsa
1/4 cup shredded fat-free or reduced-fat Cheddar cheese

COOK'S TIP

You can wrap each filled tortilla in plastic wrap as much as three days before using. Reheat one wrap (still in plastic wrap) in the microwave on 100 percent power (high) for 30 seconds to 1 minute.

1 Preheat the oven to 300°F.

2 Heat a medium nonstick skillet over medium-high heat. Cook the sausage for 6 to 8 minutes, or until cooked through, stirring to break up the meat. Pour into a colander and rinse under hot water to remove excess fat. Drain well. Set aside. Wipe the skillet with paper towels.

3 Wrap the tortillas in aluminum foil. Warm in the oven for 10 minutes.

4 Meanwhile, lightly spray the skillet with vegetable oil spray (being careful not to spray near a gas flame). Reduce the heat to medium and cook the corn for 4 to 5 minutes, or until warmed through, stirring occasionally.

5 Stir in the egg substitute and chili powder. Cook for 3 to 4 minutes, or until cooked through, stirring occasionally. Stir in the cooked sausage.

6 To assemble, spoon 1/2 cup egg mixture down the middle of each tortilla. Top each with 1 tablespoon salsa and 1 tablespoon cheese. Fold the bottom, then the sides, then the top of each tortilla toward the center.

EXCHANGES

1 1/2 Starch
1 Lean Meat

Calories	170
Calories from Fat	29
Total Fat	3 g
Saturated Fat	0.5 g
Polyunsaturated Fat	1.5 g
Monounsaturated Fat	0.6 g
Cholesterol	11 mg
Sodium	349 mg
Total Carbohydrate	26 g
Dietary Fiber	3 g
Sugars	2 g
Protein	12 g

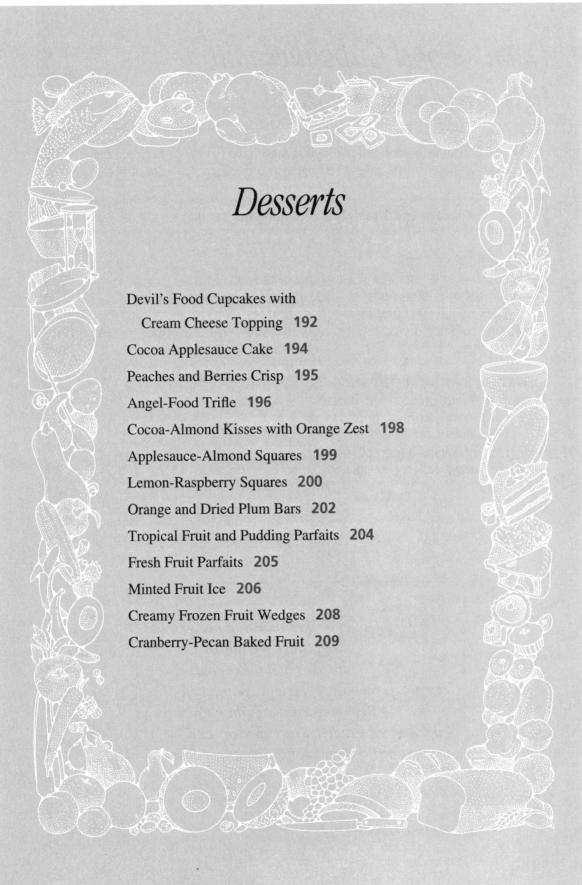

Desserts

Devil's Food Cupcakes with Cream Cheese Topping

If you love chocolate and cheesecake, you won't have to choose between them with these doubly delicious little cakes. They give you the decadent taste of both.

Serves 24; 1 cupcake and 1 tablespoon topping per serving

Vegetable oil spray
18.25-ounce package devil's food cake mix
Whites of 6 large eggs, or egg substitute equivalent to 3 eggs
2 2.25-ounce jars baby food pureed carrots
1 1/3 cups cold coffee, or 1 1/3 cups water and 1 1/4 teaspoons instant coffee granules

CREAM CHEESE TOPPING
4 ounces light tub cream cheese
3 tablespoons confectioners' sugar
2 tablespoons fat-free milk
1/2 teaspoon vanilla extract
1 cup frozen fat-free or light whipped topping, thawed

> **COOK'S TIP**
>
> *If this recipe makes more cupcakes than you need right away, store the unfrosted cupcakes and the topping in separate airtight containers. Refrigerate the topping. Frost the cupcakes as needed. The cupcakes and topping will stay fresh for about five days.*

1 Preheat the oven to 325°F. Lightly spray two 12-cup nonstick muffin pans with vegetable oil spray.

2 In a large mixing bowl, stir together the cake mix, egg whites, carrots, and coffee. Using an electric mixer, beat on low speed for 30 seconds to blend slightly. Increase the speed to medium and beat for 2 minutes. Spoon the batter into the muffin cups.

3 Bake for 20 minutes, or until a wooden toothpick inserted in the center comes out clean. Put the pans on cooling racks and let stand for 15 minutes. Remove the cupcakes from the pans and let cool completely.

4 Meanwhile, in a medium mixing bowl, combine the cream cheese, confectioners' sugar, milk, and vanilla. Using an electric mixer, beat on medium speed until smooth.

5 Using a rubber spatula, fold in the whipped topping. Cover and refrigerate until needed. Top each cooled cupcake with 1 tablespoon topping.

EXCHANGES

1 1/2 Carbohydrate

Calories 110
Calories from Fat 18
Total Fat..............................2 g
Saturated Fat ....0.9 g
Polyunsaturated Fat ....0.0 g
Monounsaturated Fat .....0.7 g
Cholesterol ....2 mg
Sodium..........................203 mg
Total Carbohydrate.........20 g
Dietary Fiber ....1 g
Sugars ....12 g
Protein ....3 g

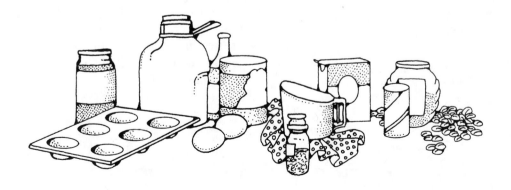

Cocoa Applesauce Cake

This cake's rich taste and moist texture come from cocoa, buttermilk, and applesauce.

Serves 24; 1 3/4-inch square per serving

Vegetable oil spray
1 1/4 cups whole-wheat pastry flour or all-purpose flour
1/4 cup uncooked regular or quick-cooking oats
1/3 cup sugar
1/3 cup unsweetened cocoa powder
1/2 tablespoon baking powder
1 teaspoon baking soda
1 cup fat-free or low-fat buttermilk
2/3 cup unsweetened applesauce
Egg substitute equivalent to 2 eggs, or 2 large eggs
3 tablespoons canola oil
1 teaspoon vanilla extract

EXCHANGES

1/2 Fat
1/2 Carbohydrate

Calories 64
  Calories from Fat 19
Total Fat............................2 g
  Saturated Fat ....0.2 g
  Polyunsaturated Fat ....0.6 g
  Monounsaturated Fat .....1.1 g
Cholesterol ....0 mg
Sodium..............................96 mg
Total Carbohydrate.........10 g
  Dietary Fiber ....1 g
  Sugars ....4 g
Protein ....2 g

1 Preheat the oven to 350°F. Lightly spray an 11 × 7 × 2-inch glass baking dish with vegetable oil spray.

2 In a medium bowl, stir together the flour, oats, sugar, cocoa, baking powder, and baking soda.

3 In a large bowl, whisk together the remaining ingredients. Stir the flour mixture into the buttermilk mixture until just combined. Spread the batter in the prepared pan.

4 Bake for 40 to 45 minutes, or until the cake springs back when gently touched in the center and a wooden toothpick inserted in the center comes out clean. Let cool completely in the pan on a cooling rack before cutting.

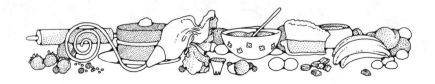

Peaches and Berries Crisp

A bounty of fruit makes this fruit crisp irresistible. It is only lightly sweetened so that the natural flavor of the fruit can come through.

Serves 8; 1/2 cup per serving

Vegetable oil spray
2 cups fresh or frozen peaches, thawed if frozen
1 cup fresh or frozen raspberries, thawed if frozen
1 cup fresh or frozen blueberries, thawed if frozen
2 tablespoons honey (1 tablespoon if using frozen peaches)
1 teaspoon lemon zest
1 teaspoon lemon juice
1/4 teaspoon ground nutmeg
1 cup uncooked quick-cooking oatmeal
1/4 cup whole-wheat flour or all-purpose flour
1/4 cup chopped walnuts
3 tablespoons light brown sugar
2 tablespoons light tub margarine, room temperature
1 teaspoon ground cinnamon

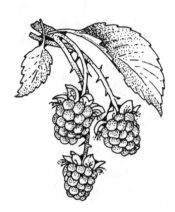

1 Preheat the oven to 350°F.

2 Lightly spray an 8-inch square baking dish with vegetable oil spray. Place the peaches, raspberries, blueberries, honey, lemon zest, lemon juice, and nutmeg in the pan, stirring gently 4 or 5 times, being careful not to break up the raspberries.

3 In a medium bowl, stir together the remaining ingredients until the margarine is distributed throughout. Sprinkle over the fruit mixture.

4 Bake for 25 to 30 minutes, or until the top is golden brown.

EXCHANGES

1/2 Fat
2 Carbohydrate

Calories	158
Calories from Fat	38
Total Fat	4 g
Saturated Fat	0.1 g
Polyunsaturated Fat	2.0 g
Monounsaturated Fat	1.4 g
Cholesterol	0 mg
Sodium	27 mg
Total Carbohydrate	29 g
Dietary Fiber	4 g
Sugars	16 g
Protein	3 g

Angel-Food Trifle

Trifle is both uptown and down home. Although it is elegant and pretty enough to serve to your company, there are enough shortcuts that you can prepare it often for family dinners, too. (See photo insert.)

Serves 12; 2/3 cup per serving

1-pound package fat-free angel food cake mix or 6-inch-diameter angel food cake
3 cups fat-free milk
2 1.5- to 1.7-ounce packages instant fat-free, sugar-free vanilla pudding mix (4-serving size)
2 cups sliced fresh strawberries
1 cup fresh blueberries
1 cup fresh raspberries
1 tablespoon sugar
1 tablespoon sweet marsala, cream sherry, or fresh orange juice
1/4 cup melted all-fruit seedless raspberry spread
1 1/2 cups frozen fat-free or light whipped topping, thawed
1/2 teaspoon vanilla extract

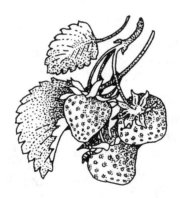

> **COOK'S TIP**
>
> *A serrated knife works well for cutting light and airy angel food cake. It is less likely to compress the cake. You can serve angel food cake plain, iced, or topped with fruit.*

1 Prepare the cake and let it cool using the package directions.

2 Meanwhile, pour the milk into a medium bowl. Add the pudding mix. Using a whisk or electric mixer, beat on low speed for 2 minutes. If not using the pudding immediately, put plastic wrap directly on it and refrigerate. (Both the cake and the pudding can be made up to a day before assembly.)

3 In a large bowl, stir together the strawberries, blueberries, raspberries, sugar, and marsala.

4 When the cake is completely cool, cut or tear enough 1/2- to 3/4-inch cubes of cake to measure 3 cups. Wrap the remaining cake in plastic wrap or aluminum foil to use another time.

5 To assemble, put half the cake cubes in a 2 1/2-quart glass bowl. Drizzle with 2 tablespoons fruit spread. Top with half the fruit mixture, followed by half the pudding. Repeat.

6 In a medium bowl, stir together the whipped topping and vanilla. Gently spread over the pudding. Cover the bowl with plastic wrap. Refrigerate until ready to serve, up to 24 hours.

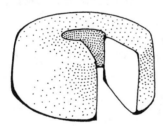

EXCHANGES

1 1/2 Carbohydrate

Calories 122
Calories from Fat 2
Total Fat............................0 g
Saturated Fat ....0.1 g
Polyunsaturated Fat ....0.1 g
Monounsaturated Fat .....0.1 g
Cholesterol ....1 mg
Sodium..........................380 mg
Total Carbohydrate........26 g
Dietary Fiber ....2 g
Sugars ....13 g
Protein ....3 g

Cocoa-Almond Kisses with Orange Zest

These little gems are crunchy on the outside and chewy on the inside. The rich taste of cocoa and almonds—plus a bit of orange zest—bursts through in every bite.

Serves 20; 2 cookies per serving

Vegetable oil spray (optional)
1/2 cup sugar
 3 tablespoons unsweetened
     cocoa powder
     Whites of 3 large eggs, room
     temperature
1/4 teaspoon cream of tartar
 1 teaspoon grated orange zest
1/2 teaspoon almond extract
1/2 cup slivered almonds, dry
     roasted and finely chopped

Room temperature egg whites will produce more volume when whipped than will egg whites straight from the refrigerator. Either take the eggs out ahead of time or briefly place them in a bowl of hot water until they come to room temperature. Adding a bit of cream of tartar to the whites also helps increase the volume. Even a single drop of egg yolk will prevent egg whites from forming peaks when beaten, so separate eggs very carefully.

1 Preheat the oven to 275°F. Lightly spray a large baking sheet with vegetable oil spray, or line it with parchment paper or aluminum foil.

2 In a small bowl, stir together the sugar and cocoa.

3 Put the egg whites and cream of tartar in a large mixing bowl. Using an electric mixer, beat at medium-high speed until foamy. Gradually add the sugar mixture to the whites. Continue to beat until the whites are shiny and form stiff peaks.

4 Using a plastic or rubber spatula, gently fold in the remaining ingredients.

5 Drop the batter by rounded teaspoons onto the prepared pan, leaving a 1-inch space between the meringues.

6 Bake for 40 minutes, or until firm. Turn the oven off and let the meringues dry in the closed oven for 30 minutes. Transfer to a cooling rack and let cool completely. Store the meringues in an airtight container.

EXCHANGES

1/2 Carbohydrate

Calories	42
Calories from Fat	16
Total Fat	2 g
Saturated Fat	0.2 g
Polyunsaturated Fat	0.4 g
Monounsaturated Fat	1.1 g
Cholesterol	0 mg
Sodium	8 mg
Total Carbohydrate	6 g
Dietary Fiber	1 g
Sugars	5 g
Protein	1 g

Applesauce-Almond Squares

Ground almonds in the dry ingredients, almond extract in the batter, and slivered almonds on the top give these tender bars a wonderfully nutty taste.

Serves 24; 1 3/4-inch square per serving

Vegetable oil spray
1 cup unsweetened applesauce
1/2 cup fat-free milk
1/3 cup fat-free or low-fat plain yogurt
3 tablespoons canola oil
Whites of 2 large eggs
1/2 teaspoon almond extract
1 cup whole-wheat pastry flour or all-purpose flour
1/4 cup plus 2 tablespoons firmly packed dark brown sugar
1/4 cup uncooked regular or quick-cooking oats
1/4 cup ground or finely chopped almonds
1/2 tablespoon baking powder
1/2 teaspoon ground cinnamon
1/4 teaspoon ground cardamom
1/8 teaspoon salt
3 tablespoons slivered almonds

COOK'S TIP *For baking, whole-wheat pastry flour is preferable to regular whole-wheat flour because the pastry flour is finer in texture and produces a tenderer finished product. You can usually find whole-wheat pastry flour with the other flour and baking ingredients in the supermarket.*

1 Preheat the oven to 350°F. Lightly spray an 11 × 7 × 2-inch baking pan with vegetable oil spray.

2 In a large bowl, whisk together the applesauce, milk, yogurt, oil, egg whites, and almond extract.

3 In a medium bowl, stir together all the remaining ingredients except the slivered almonds. Stir the flour mixture into the applesauce mixture until just combined. Spread the batter in the baking pan. Sprinkle with the slivered almonds.

4 Bake for 35 to 38 minutes, or until a wooden toothpick inserted in the center comes out clean. Let cool in the pan on a cooling rack.

EXCHANGES

1/2 Fat
1/2 Carbohydrate

Calories 74
  Calories from Fat 28
Total Fat..............................3 g
  Saturated Fat ....0.2 g
  Polyunsaturated Fat ....0.9 g
  Monounsaturated Fat .....1.8 g
Cholesterol ....0 mg
Sodium............................46 mg
Total Carbohydrate.........10 g
  Dietary Fiber ....1 g
  Sugars ....5 g
Protein ....2 g

Lemon-Raspberry Squares

These tangy bars are loaded with the sweet-tart taste of fresh lemon and raspberries. Serve them as is or with a dusting of confectioners' sugar and grated lemon zest.

Serves 24; 1 3/4-inch square per serving

Vegetable oil spray
1 medium lemon
1 cup whole-wheat pastry flour or all-purpose flour
1/3 cup regular or quick-cooking oats
1/3 cup yellow cornmeal
1/4 cup plus 2 tablespoons sugar
1/2 tablespoon baking powder
1/2 teaspoon baking soda
1/2 teaspoon ground cardamom
1/4 teaspoon cinnamon
1 cup fat-free or low-fat buttermilk
2/3 cup unsweetened applesauce
3 tablespoons canola oil
Egg substitute equivalent to 2 eggs, or 2 large eggs
1 1/2 cups fresh raspberries
1 to 2 tablespoons sifted confectioners' sugar (optional)
Grated lemon zest (optional)

COOK'S TIP

Cornmeal is used in place of some of the all-purpose flour in many Italian baked desserts. It adds a special texture and taste to the finished product.

1 Preheat the oven to 350°F. Lightly spray an 11 × 7 × 2-inch glass baking dish with vegetable oil spray.

2 Grate all the lemon zest. Put 1 teaspoon lemon zest in a medium bowl. Set the rest aside for the topping. Squeeze 2 tablespoons juice from the lemon. Set aside.

3 Stir the flour, oats, cornmeal, sugar, baking powder, baking soda, cardamom, and cinnamon into the bowl with the lemon zest.

4 In a large bowl, whisk together the buttermilk, applesauce, oil, egg substitute, and lemon juice.

5 Stir the flour mixture into the buttermilk mixture. Gently fold in the raspberries. Spread the batter in the baking dish.

6 Bake for 50 to 55 minutes, or until the top is springy to the touch and a wooden toothpick inserted in the center comes out clean. Let cool completely in the pan on a cooling rack. Sprinkle with the confectioners' sugar and reserved lemon zest.

EXCHANGES

1 Carbohydrate

Calories 69
Calories from Fat 19
Total Fat .... 2 g
Saturated Fat .... 0.1 g
Polyunsaturated Fat .... 0.6 g
Monounsaturated Fat ..... 1.0 g
Cholesterol .... 0 mg
Sodium .... 70 mg
Total Carbohydrate .... 11 g
Dietary Fiber .... 2 g
Sugars .... 5 g
Protein .... 2 g

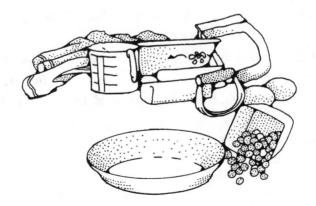

Orange and Dried Plum Bars

These squares, with their thin layer of tasty dried plum butter, are a delightful snack or dessert. Make two batches at the same time, doubling the ingredients, using the oven just once, and freezing a batch for later.

Serves 24; 1 3/4-inch square per serving

    Vegetable oil spray
1 cup regular or quick-cooking oats
1 cup whole-wheat pastry flour or all-purpose flour
1/4 cup sugar
1/2 teaspoon ground cardamom
1/4 teaspoon ground nutmeg
1/4 teaspoon baking soda
    Whites of 2 large eggs
1 orange
3 tablespoons canola oil
1 1/2 cups fruit butter, such as dried plum or apple

> **COOK'S TIP**
>
> *Pastry flour is a low-gluten flour milled from soft winter wheat. Some cake, piecrust, and muffin recipes (but not breads) call for pastry flour because it produces a finer, lighter texture than all-purpose flour. Whole-wheat pastry flour utilizes all the kernel (bran and germ), making it very nutritious. Whole-wheat pastry flour is denser than regular pastry flour and imparts a rustic, earthy quality to the finished product. Look near the other flours and baking ingredients in supermarkets for these products.*

1 Preheat the oven to 350°F. Lightly spray an 8-inch square baking pan with vegetable oil spray.

2 In a medium bowl, stir together the oats, flour, sugar, cardamom, nutmeg, and baking soda.

3 In a small bowl, using a fork, lightly beat the egg whites.

4 Grate 2 teaspoons zest from the orange. Set aside. Squeeze 2 tablespoons juice from the orange. Stir the orange juice and oil into the egg whites.

5 Add the egg white mixture to the oat mixture, stirring until the combined mixture holds together. Press three-fourths of the mixture into the baking pan.

6 In a medium bowl, stir together the fruit butter and orange zest. Using a rubber scraper, spread the fruit mixture over the oat mixture. Sprinkle with the remaining oat mixture.

7 Bake for 30 to 35 minutes, or until the top is golden brown. Let cool completely in the pan on a cooling rack before cutting.

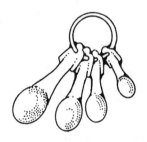

EXCHANGES

1 Carbohydrate

Calories	86
Calories from Fat	18
Total Fat	2 g
Saturated Fat	0.2 g
Polyunsaturated Fat	0.6 g
Monounsaturated Fat	1.1 g
Cholesterol	0 mg
Sodium	19 mg
Total Carbohydrate	16 g
Dietary Fiber	1 g
Sugars	8 g
Protein	1 g

Tropical Fruit and Pudding Parfaits

Flavors of the tropics, including mango, pineapple, and coconut, harmonize well with thick, creamy pudding for a cool and refreshing summer dessert.

Serves 6; 1 cup per serving

2 cups fat-free milk
    1-ounce package (4-serving size) fat-free, sugar-free instant vanilla pudding mix or 3.4-ounce package regular instant vanilla pudding mix
1/2 teaspoon coconut extract
1/4 teaspoon ground ginger (optional)
1 cup frozen fat-free or light whipped topping, thawed
1 cup canned pineapple tidbits in their own juice, drained
1 medium mango, diced, or 1 cup diced bottled mango
1 medium banana, thinly sliced
1 tablespoon light brown sugar
1 teaspoon orange zest
1/4 teaspoon ground nutmeg
1/2 cup crushed reduced-fat vanilla wafer cookies (about 12)

1 In a medium bowl, whisk together the milk, pudding mix, coconut extract, and ginger for 2 minutes.

2 Gently whisk in the whipped topping. Refrigerate for 5 minutes.

3 Meanwhile, in a medium bowl, stir together the remaining ingredients except the cookie crumbs.

4 To assemble, spoon about 1/4 cup fruit into each parfait or wine glass. Spoon 1/4 cup pudding over each serving. Sprinkle each with about 2 teaspoons crushed cookies. Repeat.

EXCHANGES

2 1/2 Carbohydrate

Calories 167
Calories from Fat 7
Total Fat...........................1 g
Saturated Fat ....0.4 g
Polyunsaturated Fat ....0.1 g
Monounsaturated Fat .....0.3 g
Cholesterol ....2 mg
Sodium...........................284 mg
Total Carbohydrate.........36 g
Dietary Fiber ....2 g
Sugars ....23 g
Protein ....3 g

Fresh Fruit Parfaits

This dessert takes full advantage of the seasonal bounty of available fruit. In winter, try apples, pears, and grapefruit and orange sections and use frozen unsweetened strawberries for the sauce.

Serves 4; 1 cup fruit and 2 tablespoons sauce per serving

SAUCE
  2 cups fresh strawberries (quartered if large)
  2 tablespoons all-fruit seedless raspberry spread
  1 tablespoon peach brandy or peach nectar
1/2 teaspoon almond extract

FRUIT
  1 cup fresh blueberries
  1 cup fresh raspberries
  1 cup sliced fresh strawberries
  1 cup chopped fresh peaches or
    nectarines

1 For the sauce, in a food processor or blender, process the ingredients until smooth, stopping the motor once or twice to scrape down the sides of the bowl. Strain the sauce through a fine-mesh sieve if you prefer a smoother texture.

2 To assemble, layer the fruit in parfait or wine glasses. Spoon 2 tablespoons sauce over each parfait.

EXCHANGES

2 Fruit

Calories	111
Calories from Fat	3
Total Fat	0 g
Saturated Fat	0.0 g
Polyunsaturated Fat	0.0 g
Monounsaturated Fat	0.0 g
Cholesterol	0 mg
Sodium	6 mg
Total Carbohydrate	27 g
Dietary Fiber	6 g
Sugars	18 g
Protein	2 g

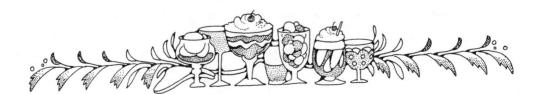

Minted Fruit Ice

This cold and refreshing dessert is bursting with fabulous fruit and a touch of aromatic fresh mint. The only difficult part about this dish is deciding whether to make it icy or to add the extra juice to make it creamy in texture.

Serves 8; 1/2 cup per serving

    1 cup pineapple juice or fresh orange juice
  1/4 cup sugar
    2 teaspoons snipped fresh mint
    1 teaspoon grated lime zest
    2 cups strawberries, quartered if large
    2 peaches or nectarines, peeled and coarsely chopped
    1 medium banana
    2 tablespoons fresh lime juice
    3 tablespoons pineapple juice or fresh orange juice (optional for creamy version)

COOK'S TIP

The easy way to get the zest from citrus fruit is to use a zester or food rasp. Zesters are tools that have small holes at one end. Pull the zester over the outer layer of the fruit to get thin strands of colored rind. Be careful to avoid grating any of the white layer, which is bitter. Rasps look and function like thin graters, usually with a handle at one end for better control, and come in various lengths. A food rasp also works well for grating ginger.

---

1 In a small nonreactive saucepan (such as stainless steel), bring the 1 cup pineapple juice, sugar, mint, and lime zest to a boil over medium heat. Boil for 1 minute. Pour into a medium bowl.

2 Fill a large bowl with ice cubes. Place the bowl with the juice mixture on the ice. Let the juice cool for 15 to 20 minutes, or until room temperature.

3 In a food processor or blender, process the remaining ingredients except the 3 tablespoons pineapple juice until smooth, stopping the motor once or twice to scrape down the sides of the bowl. With the motor running, pour the juice mixture through the feed tube. Process until blended.

4 Pour the mixture into a metal 11 × 7 × 2-inch pan. Cover the pan with aluminum foil or plastic wrap. Freeze for 2 to 3 hours, or until the edges are hard.

5 Break up the fruit ice in the pan and transfer it back to the food processor. Process the mixture to the consistency of crushed ice. Or add the 3 tablespoons pineapple juice and process for 2 minutes, or until the texture is creamy.

6 Serve immediately or transfer to an airtight container and freeze again. Remove from the freezer 15 to 20 minutes before serving.

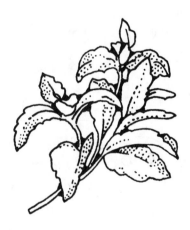

EXCHANGES

(icy version; the creamy version
has 3 more calories and
1 more carb gram)

1 1/2 Fruit

Calories 83
Calories from Fat 0
Total Fat............................0 g
Saturated Fat ....0 g
Polyunsaturated Fat ....0 g
Monounsaturated Fat ....0 g
Cholesterol ....0 mg
Sodium..............................1 mg
Total Carbohydrate.........21 g
Dietary Fiber ....2 g
Sugars ....18 g
Protein ....1 g

Creamy Frozen Fruit Wedges

This extremely easy, make-ahead dessert is perfect for the little kid in each of us. Simply toss a few ingredients together and pop the pie in the freezer. If you just can't wait, you can even eat it unfrozen, like pudding.

Serves 8; 1 wedge per serving

    1   pound frozen unsweetened whole strawberries
1 1/2   cups fat-free or low-fat vanilla yogurt
        8-ounce can crushed pineapple in its own juice, drained
    2   cups frozen fat-free or light whipped topping, thawed

1   In a medium bowl, stir together the strawberries, yogurt, and pineapple.

2   Gently fold in the whipped topping. Spoon the mixture into a 9-inch pie pan. Cover with plastic wrap and freeze for 4 hours, or until firm.

3   Remove the pie from the freezer about 15 minutes before serving to let it thaw slightly. Cut into wedges.

When you need a really quick dessert, substitute fresh berries for the frozen variety, combine the ingredients without freezing, and serve in chilled wine goblets.

COOK'S TIP

EXCHANGES

1 Carbohydrate

Calories 84
 Calories from Fat 0
Total Fat............................0 g
 Saturated Fat ....0 g
 Polyunsaturated Fat ....0 g
 Monounsaturated Fat ....0 g
Cholesterol ....1 mg
Sodium...........................38 mg
Total Carbohydrate.........18 g
 Dietary Fiber ....1 g
 Sugars ....11 g
Protein ....2 g

Cranberry-Pecan Baked Fruit

Fresh fruit is baked upside down over pecans, dried cranberries, and honey, then turned over and filled with the mixture and its roasted, concentrated flavors. It's perfect for dessert any season of the year.

Serves 4; 2 peach halves and 2 tablespoons cranberry mixture per serving

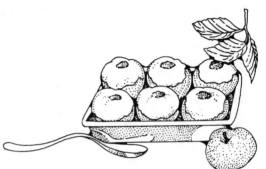

Vegetable oil spray
1 1/2 tablespoons honey
4 medium peaches, nectarines, or pears, halved, pitted, and pierced several times with a fork
1/3 cup dried cranberries
3 tablespoons pecan pieces
2 teaspoons light tub margarine
1/2 teaspoon grated peeled gingerroot

1 Preheat the oven to 350°F.

2 Lightly spray a 9-inch pie pan with vegetable oil spray. Pour the honey into the pie pan. Heat in the oven for 2 minutes, or until slightly runny. Remove the pan from the oven. Tilt the pan so the honey lightly coats the bottom.

3 Sprinkle the cranberries and pecans evenly in the pan. Place the peaches with the cut side down over the cranberry mixture. (Some of the cranberry mixture may not be covered.) Cover the pan with aluminum foil. Bake for 30 minutes, or until tender.

4 Arrange the peaches with the cut side up on a serving plate. Stir the margarine and gingerroot into the pan juices. Spoon over the peaches. Serve warm or at room temperature.

EXCHANGES

2 Fruit
1 Fat

Calories 164
  Calories from Fat 45
Total Fat..............................5 g
  Saturated Fat ....0.3 g
  Polyunsaturated Fat ....1.4 g
  Monounsaturated Fat .....2.8 g
Cholesterol ....0 mg
Sodium.............................16 mg
Total Carbohydrate.........31 g
  Dietary Fiber ....4 g
  Sugars ....26 g
Protein ....2 g

Alphabetical Index

Subject Index

Appetizers

Boneless Buffalo Wings, 12
Dijon Dip with Tarragon, 5
Layered Fiesta Bean Dip, 2
Peach and Pineapple Dip, 6
Savory Stuffed Eggs, 8
Skewered Antipasto, 7
Spinach and Artichoke Dip, 3
Stuffed Mushrooms with Ham and
    Vegetables, 10
Triple-Duty Ranch Dip with Dill, 4

Beef

Company Roast Tenderloin, 104
Fabulous Fajitas, 108
Grilled Meat Loaf, 120
Grilled Sirloin with Tapenade, 113
Mexican-Style Stuffed Bell Peppers, 116
Mushroom-Smothered Cube Steak, 106
Roast Sirloin and Vegetable Supper, 115
Sassy Beef and Onion Kebabs, 114
Slow-Cooker Mediterranean Pot Roast, 105
Slow-Cooker Swiss Steak, 112
Spicy Orange Flank Steak, 110
Swedish Meatballs, 118
Tex-Mex Chili Bowl, 111

Beverages

Chocolate-Mocha Cooler, 13

Breads (*also see* Cakes; Muffins)

Rosemary and Dill Quick Bread, 180

Breakfasts

Apple Pie Breakfast Parfaits, 185
Apricot and Apple Granola, 184
French Toast Casserole with Honey-
    Glazed Fruit, 186
Ham-and-Swiss Breakfast Casserole, 187

Ham and Broccoli Frittata, 127
Southwestern Breakfast Tortilla Wrap, 188

Cakes

Angel Food Trifle, 196
Apple Crumble Coffee Cake, 182
Cocoa Applesauce Cake, 194
Devil's Food Cupcakes with Cream
    Cheese Topping, 192

Chicken

Baked Chicken Parmesan, 87
Boneless Buffalo Wings, 12
Cheese-Filled Oven-Fried Chicken, 88
Chicken and Asparagus Toss, 89
Chicken and Noodles with Alfredo-Style
    Sauce, 92
Chicken Antipasto Salad, 48
Chicken Pot Pie, 96
Chicken Stir-Fry with Snow Peas and
    Mixed Bell Peppers, 84
Chicken with Country Gravy, 90
Citrus Chicken, 94
Creole Drums, 95
Oven-Fried Sesame-Ginger Chicken, 86
Roast Chicken Breasts with Vegetable
    Medley, 82
Seared Chicken with Strawberry Salsa, 91
Skillet Chicken with Lime Barbecue
    Sauce, 93
Tex-Mex Chicken Fingers, 85

Desserts (*also see* Cakes)

Angel-Food Trifle, 196
Applesauce-Almond Squares, 199
Cocoa-Almond Kisses with Orange Zest,
    198
Cranberry-Pecan Baked Fruit, 209
Creamy Frozen Fruit Wedges, 208
Fresh Fruit Parfaits, 205

Tuna-Macaroni Casserole with Tomatoes
and Chickpeas, 69

Shrimp

Lemony Shrimp Salad, 50
Parsley Pesto Shrimp, 75
Deep-South Shrimp Gumbo, 79

Soups

Broccoli Cheese Soup, 16
Corn and Ham Chowder, 25
Creamy Caramelized Onion Soup, 18
Deep-South Shrimp Gumbo, 79
Home-Style Vegetable Beef Soup, 23
Italian Lentil Soup, 30
Loaded Baked Potato Soup, 20
Mushroom and Barley Stew, 26
Pork, Barley, and Vegetable Stew, 24
Split Pea and Lima Bean Soup with
Chicken, 22
Tomato Basil Bisque, 17
Vegetable Stew with Fresh Rosemary, 28

Turkey

Cranberry-Pecan Turkey Salad, 49
Roast Turkey with Orange-Spice Rub, 97
Stir-Fry Turkey Strips with Broccoli,
Green Onions, and Water
Chestnuts, 100
Turkey Chili, 102
Turkey Loaf, 99
Turkey Marsala, 98

Vegetables

Acorn Squash Filled with Dried Apricots
and Plums, 171
Asian Broccoli with Pecans, 159
Brown-Sugar-and-Spice Sweet Potatoes,
167
Down-Home Greens, 162

Italian Skillet Spinach, 170
Lemon-Mint Sugar Snaps, 164
Mediterranean Couscous with Capers, 161
Mediterranean Zucchini, 174
Mushrooms Marinated in Lime and Soy
Sauce, 163
Nutmeg-Spiced Vegetable Medley, 177
Pecan-Roasted Asparagus, 158
Red Pepper Pilaf, 168
Red Potatoes Parmesan, 165
Roasted Green Beans Dijon, 160
Scalloped Potatoes, 166
Tarragon Tomatoes, 175
Thyme-Tinged Squash, 172
Toasted-Almond Rice and Peas, 169
Veggie Stir-Fry, Mexican Style, 176
Zucchini Sticks, 173

Vegetarian Entrées

Bean and Cheese Tostadas, 145
Chili-Stuffed Potato Boats, 156
Chunky Vegetable and Egg Salad
Sandwiches, 148
Crustless Asparagus and Tomato Quiche,
149
Eggplant Ricotta Lasagna, 134
Italian Eggplant, 150
Lentil Stew with Vegetarian Hot Dogs,
154
Lentils with Brown Rice and Mushrooms,
142
Mexican Yellow Rice and Black Beans,
136
Middle Eastern Brown Rice and Pine
Nuts, 153
Red Beans and Brown Rice, 137
Roasted-Veggie Pizza on a Phyllo Crust,
130
Six-Ingredient Lasagna, 133
Skillet-Roasted Veggie Scramble, 146

About the American Diabetes Association

The American Diabetes Association is the nation's leading voluntary health organization supporting diabetes research, information, and advocacy. Its mission is to prevent and cure diabetes and to improve the lives of all people affected by diabetes. The American Diabetes Association is the leading publisher of comprehensive diabetes information. Its huge library of practical and authoritative books for people with diabetes covers every aspect of self-care—cooking and nutrition, fitness, weight control, medications, complications, emotional issues, and general self-care.

To order American Diabetes Association books: Call 1-800-232-6733.
Or log on to http://store.diabetes.org

To join the American Diabetes Association: Call 1-800-806-7801.
www.diabetes.org/membership

For more information about diabetes or ADA programs and services: Call 1-800-342-2383.
E-mail: Customerservice@diabetes.org or log on to www.diabetes.org

To locate an ADA/NCQA Recognized Provider of quality diabetes care in your area:
www.ncqa.org/dprp

To find an ADA Recognized Education Program in your area: Call 1-888-232-0822.
www.diabetes.org/recognition/education.asp

To join the fight to increase funding for diabetes research, end discrimination, and improve insurance coverage: Call 1-800-342-2383. www.diabetes.org/advocacy

To find out how you can get involved with the programs in your community:
Call 1-800-342-2383. See below for program Web addresses.

- American Diabetes Month: educational activities aimed at those diagnosed with diabetes—month of November. www.diabetes.org/ADM
- American Diabetes Alert: annual public awareness campaign to find the undiagnosed—held the fourth Tuesday in March. www.diabetes.org/alert
- The Diabetes Assistance & Resources Program (DAR): diabetes awareness program targeted to the Latino community. www.diabetes.org/DAR
- African American Program: diabetes awareness program targeted to the African American community. www.diabetes.org/africanamerican
- Awakening the Spirit: Pathways to Diabetes Prevention & Control: diabetes awareness program targeted to the Native American community. www.diabetes.org/awakening

To find out about an important research project regarding type 2 diabetes:
www.diabetes.org/ada/research.asp

To obtain information on making a planned gift or charitable bequest: Call 1-888-700-7029.
www.diabetes.org/ada/plan.asp

To make a donation or memorial contribution: Call 1-800-342-2383.
www.diabetes.org/ada/cont.asp

About the American Heart Association

The American Heart Association is the nation's premier authority on heart health, with a best-selling library of cookbooks and health guides. The American Heart Association and the American Stroke Association work every day to advance groundbreaking research, spread lifesaving knowledge, and help all Americans live longer, healthier lives. In communities throughout America, we help safeguard people of all ages from the devastation of heart disease and stroke.

The American Heart Association is headquartered in Dallas, Texas, with affiliates that serve the entire United States.

American Heart Association cookbooks are available wherever books are sold.

For information about heart disease and the American Heart Association:
Call 1-800-AHA-USA1 (1-800-242-8721) or visit americanheart.org.
You can also write to American Heart Association, 7272 Greenville Avenue, Dallas, Texas 75231-4596.

To join or make a donation to the Association:
Call 1-800-AHA-USA1 (1-800-242-8721) or visit americanheart.org.
You can also write to American Heart Association, 7272 Greenville Avenue, Dallas, Texas 75231-4596.

To find out how to get involved in the Association's many programs:
Call 1-800-AHA-USA1 (1-800-242-8721) or visit americanheart.org for information about:

- Heart Walk
- Cholesterol Low Down™
- Heart Of Diabetes: Understanding Insulin Resistance[SM]
- Jump Rope For Heart and Hoops For Heart

Call 1-888-MY-HEART (1-888-694-3278) or visit americanheart.org for these programs for women:

- Go Red For Women[SM]
- Choose To Move[SM]
- Simple Solutions

For information about stroke and the American Stroke Association:
Call 1-888-4-STROKE (1-888-478-7653) or visit strokeassociation.org.
You can also write to American Stroke Association, 7272 Greenville Avenue, Dallas, Texas 75231-4596.